12-Week Fasting Journal

A Guided 12-Week Tracker for Fasting, Energy, Hunger, and Recovery

Nathan Reed

PERENNIAL PUBLISHING

Published by Perennial Publishing

Paperback ISBN: 978-1-971996-72-1

Contents

Disclaimer

This journal is provided for educational and personal tracking purposes only. It is not medical advice, nutritional counseling, a fasting protocol, a treatment plan, or a substitute for guidance from a qualified healthcare professional.

Fasting may not be appropriate for everyone. Before beginning or extending any fasting practice, consult a qualified healthcare professional, especially if you are pregnant, breastfeeding, underweight, under medical care, taking prescription medication, managing diabetes or blood sugar concerns, managing blood pressure concerns, have a history of eating disorders or disordered eating, have a diagnosed medical condition, or are unsure whether fasting is appropriate for you.

The pages in this journal are intended to help you record observations such as fasting windows, eating windows, hunger, energy, cravings, sleep, electrolytes, fluids, stress, and recovery. These entries are not diagnostic measurements and should not be used to self-diagnose, treat, prevent, or cure any disease or medical condition.

Do not force a fast to match this journal. If you experience concerning symptoms, severe weakness, dizziness, fainting, confusion, chest pain, persistent vomiting, abnormal heart symptoms, or any other serious or unusual reaction, stop fasting and seek appropriate medical help.

Use this journal as an observation tool. Your health, safety, and medical context should always come before completing a fasting window, filling out a tracker, or reaching a planned duration.

Before the Fast

Fasting Stability Journal

How to Use This Tracker

① Before You Begin

- Fill out the prep page.
- Note your planned fasting window.
- Have needed items available.
- Note context such as sleep, stress, training, travel, or illness.

② Each Day

- Complete the Daily Tracking Day spread.
- Record fasting window and eating window.
- Record morning stats and daily signals.
- Add electrolyte / fluid notes and observations.

③ At the End of the Cycle

- Complete the Weekly Review and pattern pages.
- Note what felt stable or unstable.
- Plan the next cycle.

④ Keep It Observational

- Use ratings as signals not grades.
- Do not force the fast to match the journal.
- Reassess if something feels off.

Quick Reminder

____

____

____

____

Fasting Stability Journal

Daily Rating Key

(1) 1–5 Scale

1	=	Very Low / Minimal
2	=	Low
3	=	Moderate
4	=	High
5	=	Very High

(2) How to Read the Scale

(+) For positive signals such as Energy and Mental Clarity, higher numbers mean more available.

(−) For pressure signals such as Hunger, Cravings, and Stress, higher numbers mean more intense.

(3) Use One Number

- Choose the number that best matches the day overall.
- Do not overthink the scale.
- Use the ratings for pattern recognition over time.

(4) Notes

Fasting Stability Journal

Fasting Cycle Prep

1 Planned Fast

Start: ____________ End: ____________ Target Duration: ____________

2 Reason for Tracking This Cycle

____

____

____

3 Items to Have Available

- ☐ Water
- ☐ Sodium / Salt
- ☐ Magnesium
- ☐ Potassium / Electrolyte Source
- ☐ Electrolytes
- ☐ Caffeine / Tea / Coffee
- ☐ Blood Glucose Meter
- ☐ Ketone Meter
- ☐ Blood Pressure Monitor
- ☐ Scale
- ☐ Notes / Symptom Log

4 Context to Watch

- ☐ Poor Sleep
- ☐ High Stress
- ☐ Heavy Training
- ☐ Travel
- ☐ Illness / Recovery
- ☐ Unusual Appetite
- ☐ Medication Considerations
- ☐ Other: ____________

5 Baseline Notes Before Starting

____

____

____

____

6 Important Signals to Monitor

____

____

____

____

Fasting Stability Journal

Cycle Start

① Cycle Start Details

Start Date: ______________________ Start Time: ______________________

Planned End Date: ______________________ Planned End Time: ______________________

Planned Duration: ____

② Fasting Experience

- [ ] Beginner
- [ ] Some Experience
- [ ] Experienced

③ Starting Baseline

Sleep Quality	1	2	3	4	5
Energy	1	2	3	4	5
Hunger	1	2	3	4	5
Stress	1	2	3	4	5

④ Current Context

Training / Activity Load: ____

Work / Schedule Load: ____

Travel / Routine Change: ____

⑤ What I Want to Observe This Cycle

____

____

____

____

⑥ Additional Notes

____

____

____

The Fast

Fasting Stability Journal

Daily Tracking Day _____

Day: ______________________ Date: ______________________

1 Fasting Window

Start: ______________ End: ______________ Total Hours: __________

2 Eating Window

Start: ______________________ End: ______________________

3 Morning Stats

Weight ______________________

Blood Glucose ______________________

Ketones ______________________

Blood Pressure ______________________

Resting Heart Rate ______________________

4 Daily Signals

Hunger	1	2	3	4	5
Cravings	1	2	3	4	5
Energy	1	2	3	4	5
Mental Clarity	1	2	3	4	5
Stress	1	2	3	4	5
Sleep Quality	1	2	3	4	5

Fasting Stability Journal

Daily Tracking Day _____

Day: ____________________ Date: ____________________

⑤ Electrolytes / Fluids

Water ____________________

Sodium ____________________

Potassium ____________________

Magnesium ____________________

Caffeine ____________________

Exercise / Sweating ____________________

⑥ Notes / Observations

____

____

____

____

____

____

⑦ What Felt Stable?

____

____

____

____

⑧ What Felt Unstable?

____

____

____

____

____

Fasting Stability Journal

Daily Tracking Day _____

Day: ____________________ Date: ____________________

1 Fasting Window

Start: ______________ End: ______________ Total Hours: __________

2 Eating Window

Start: ____________________ End: ____________________

3 Morning Stats

Weight ____________________

Blood Glucose ____________________

Ketones ____________________

Blood Pressure ____________________

Resting Heart Rate ____________________

4 Daily Signals

Hunger	1	2	3	4	5
Cravings	1	2	3	4	5
Energy	1	2	3	4	5
Mental Clarity	1	2	3	4	5
Stress	1	2	3	4	5
Sleep Quality	1	2	3	4	5

Fasting Stability Journal

Daily Tracking Day _____

Day: ______________ Date: ______________

5 Electrolytes / Fluids

Water ______________

Sodium ______________

Potassium ______________

Magnesium ______________

Caffeine ______________

Exercise / Sweating ______________

6 Notes / Observations

7 What Felt Stable?

8 What Felt Unstable?

Fasting Stability Journal

Daily Tracking Day _____

Day: ______________________ Date: ______________________

1 Fasting Window

Start: ______________ End: ______________ Total Hours: __________

2 Eating Window

Start: ______________________ End: ______________________

3 Morning Stats

Weight ______________________

Blood Glucose ______________________

Ketones ______________________

Blood Pressure ______________________

Resting Heart Rate ______________________

4 Daily Signals

Hunger	1	2	3	4	5
Cravings	1	2	3	4	5
Energy	1	2	3	4	5
Mental Clarity	1	2	3	4	5
Stress	1	2	3	4	5
Sleep Quality	1	2	3	4	5

Fasting Stability Journal

Daily Tracking Day ______

Day: ____________________ Date: ____________________

5 Electrolytes / Fluids

Water ____________________

Sodium ____________________

Potassium ____________________

Magnesium ____________________

Caffeine ____________________

Exercise / Sweating ____________________

6 Notes / Observations

____

____

____

____

____

____

7 What Felt Stable?

____

____

____

____

8 What Felt Unstable?

____

____

____

____

____

Fasting Stability Journal

Daily Tracking Day _____

Day: ______________________ Date: ______________________

① Fasting Window

Start: ______________ End: ______________ Total Hours: __________

② Eating Window

Start: ______________________ End: ______________________

③ Morning Stats

Weight ______________________

Blood Glucose ______________________

Ketones ______________________

Blood Pressure ______________________

Resting Heart Rate ______________________

④ Daily Signals

Hunger	1	2	3	4	5
Cravings	1	2	3	4	5
Energy	1	2	3	4	5
Mental Clarity	1	2	3	4	5
Stress	1	2	3	4	5
Sleep Quality	1	2	3	4	5

Fasting Stability Journal

Daily Tracking Day ____

Day: ______________ Date: ______________

(5) Electrolytes / Fluids

Water ______________

Sodium ______________

Potassium ______________

Magnesium ______________

Caffeine ______________

Exercise / Sweating ______________

(6) Notes / Observations

____

____

____

____

____

____

(7) What Felt Stable?

____

____

____

____

(8) What Felt Unstable?

____

____

____

____

____

Fasting Stability Journal

Daily Tracking Day _____

Day: ____________________ Date: ____________________

① Fasting Window

Start: ______________ End: ______________ Total Hours: __________

② Eating Window

Start: ____________________ End: ____________________

③ Morning Stats

Weight ____________________

Blood Glucose ____________________

Ketones ____________________

Blood Pressure ____________________

Resting Heart Rate ____________________

④ Daily Signals

Hunger	1	2	3	4	5
Cravings	1	2	3	4	5
Energy	1	2	3	4	5
Mental Clarity	1	2	3	4	5
Stress	1	2	3	4	5
Sleep Quality	1	2	3	4	5

Fasting Stability Journal

Daily Tracking Day _____

Day: ____________________ Date: ____________________

(5) Electrolytes / Fluids

Water ____________________

Sodium ____________________

Potassium ____________________

Magnesium ____________________

Caffeine ____________________

Exercise / Sweating ____________________

(6) Notes / Observations

____

____

____

____

____

____

(7) What Felt Stable?

____

____

____

____

(8) What Felt Unstable?

____

____

____

____

____

Fasting Stability Journal

Daily Tracking Day _____

Day: ______________________ Date: ______________________

1 Fasting Window

Start: ______________ End: ______________ Total Hours: __________

2 Eating Window

Start: ______________________ End: ______________________

3 Morning Stats

Weight ______________________

Blood Glucose ______________________

Ketones ______________________

Blood Pressure ______________________

Resting Heart Rate ______________________

4 Daily Signals

Hunger	1	2	3	4	5
Cravings	1	2	3	4	5
Energy	1	2	3	4	5
Mental Clarity	1	2	3	4	5
Stress	1	2	3	4	5
Sleep Quality	1	2	3	4	5

Fasting Stability Journal

Daily Tracking Day _____

Day: ____________________ Date: ____________________

⑤ Electrolytes / Fluids

Water ____________________

Sodium ____________________

Potassium ____________________

Magnesium ____________________

Caffeine ____________________

Exercise / Sweating ____________________

⑥ Notes / Observations

⑦ What Felt Stable?

⑧ What Felt Unstable?

Fasting Stability Journal

Daily Tracking Day _____

Day: ____________________ Date: ____________________

1 Fasting Window

Start: ______________ End: ______________ Total Hours: __________

2 Eating Window

Start: ____________________ End: ____________________

3 Morning Stats

Weight ____________________

Blood Glucose ______________

Ketones ____________________

Blood Pressure ______________

Resting Heart Rate ____________

4 Daily Signals

Hunger	1	2	3	4	5
Cravings	1	2	3	4	5
Energy	1	2	3	4	5
Mental Clarity	1	2	3	4	5
Stress	1	2	3	4	5
Sleep Quality	1	2	3	4	5

Fasting Stability Journal

Daily Tracking Day _____

Day: ____________________ Date: ____________________

(5) Electrolytes / Fluids

Water ____________________

Sodium ____________________

Potassium ____________________

Magnesium ____________________

Caffeine ____________________

Exercise / Sweating ____________________

(6) Notes / Observations

____

____

____

____

____

____

(7) What Felt Stable?

____

____

____

____

(8) What Felt Unstable?

____

____

____

____

____

Fasting Stability Journal

Weekly Review

① Cycle Review

Cycle Start: ____________ Cycle End: ____________ Days Tracked: ________

② Review Highlights

Most Stable Day: ____________________

Most Unstable Day: ____________________

Most Common Fasting Window: ____________________

Most Difficult Time of Day: ____________________

③ Signal Trends

Hunger	1	2	3	4	5
Cravings	1	2	3	4	5
Energy	1	2	3	4	5
Sleep	1	2	3	4	5
Stress	1	2	3	4	5

④ Main Patterns Noticed

____

____

____

____

⑤ What to Watch Next Cycle

____

____

____

____

____

Fasting Stability Journal

Daily Tracking Day _____

Day: ______________________ Date: ______________________

1 Fasting Window

Start: ______________ End: ______________ Total Hours: __________

2 Eating Window

Start: ______________________ End: ______________________

3 Morning Stats

Weight ______________________

Blood Glucose ______________________

Ketones ______________________

Blood Pressure ______________________

Resting Heart Rate ______________________

4 Daily Signals

Hunger	1	2	3	4	5
Cravings	1	2	3	4	5
Energy	1	2	3	4	5
Mental Clarity	1	2	3	4	5
Stress	1	2	3	4	5
Sleep Quality	1	2	3	4	5

Fasting Stability Journal

Daily Tracking Day _____

Day: ____________________ Date: ____________________

(5) Electrolytes / Fluids

Water ____________________

Sodium ____________________

Potassium ____________________

Magnesium ____________________

Caffeine ____________________

Exercise / Sweating ____________________

(6) Notes / Observations

(7) What Felt Stable?

(8) What Felt Unstable?

Fasting Stability Journal

Daily Tracking Day _____

Day: ______________________ Date: ______________________

1 Fasting Window

Start: ______________ End: ______________ Total Hours: __________

2 Eating Window

Start: ____________________ End: ________________

3 Morning Stats

Weight ____________________

Blood Glucose ________________

Ketones ____________________

Blood Pressure ________________

Resting Heart Rate ______________

4 Daily Signals

Hunger	1	2	3	4	5
Cravings	1	2	3	4	5
Energy	1	2	3	4	5
Mental Clarity	1	2	3	4	5
Stress	1	2	3	4	5
Sleep Quality	1	2	3	4	5

Fasting Stability Journal

Daily Tracking Day _____

Day: ____________ Date: ____________

5 Electrolytes / Fluids

Water ____________

Sodium ____________

Potassium ____________

Magnesium ____________

Caffeine ____________

Exercise / Sweating ____________

6 Notes / Observations

7 What Felt Stable?

8 What Felt Unstable?

Fasting Stability Journal

Daily Tracking Day ____

Day: ______________________ Date: ______________________

① Fasting Window

Start: ________________ End: ______________ Total Hours: __________

② Eating Window

Start: ______________________ End: __________________

③ Morning Stats

Weight ____________________

Blood Glucose ______________

Ketones ___________________

Blood Pressure ______________

Resting Heart Rate ___________

④ Daily Signals

Hunger	1	2	3	4	5
Cravings	1	2	3	4	5
Energy	1	2	3	4	5
Mental Clarity	1	2	3	4	5
Stress	1	2	3	4	5
Sleep Quality	1	2	3	4	5

Fasting Stability Journal

Daily Tracking Day _____

Day: ____________________ Date: ____________________

5 Electrolytes / Fluids

Water ____________________

Sodium ____________________

Potassium ____________________

Magnesium ____________________

Caffeine ____________________

Exercise / Sweating ____________________

6 Notes / Observations

____

____

____

____

____

____

7 What Felt Stable?

____

____

____

____

8 What Felt Unstable?

____

____

____

____

____

Fasting Stability Journal

Daily Tracking Day _____

Day: ______________________ Date: ______________________

1 Fasting Window

Start: ______________ End: ______________ Total Hours: __________

2 Eating Window

Start: ______________________ End: ____________________

3 Morning Stats

Weight ______________________

Blood Glucose ________________

Ketones _____________________

Blood Pressure ________________

Resting Heart Rate ______________

4 Daily Signals

Hunger	1	2	3	4	5
Cravings	1	2	3	4	5
Energy	1	2	3	4	5
Mental Clarity	1	2	3	4	5
Stress	1	2	3	4	5
Sleep Quality	1	2	3	4	5

Fasting Stability Journal

Daily Tracking Day _____

Day: ____________________ Date: ____________________

5 Electrolytes / Fluids

Water ____________________

Sodium ____________________

Potassium ____________________

Magnesium ____________________

Caffeine ____________________

Exercise / Sweating ____________________

6 Notes / Observations

7 What Felt Stable?

8 What Felt Unstable?

Fasting Stability Journal

Daily Tracking Day ____

Day: ______________________ Date: ______________________

1 Fasting Window

Start: ______________ End: ______________ Total Hours: ________

2 Eating Window

Start: ______________________ End: ______________________

3 Morning Stats

Weight ______________________

Blood Glucose ______________________

Ketones ______________________

Blood Pressure ______________________

Resting Heart Rate ______________________

4 Daily Signals

Hunger	1	2	3	4	5
Cravings	1	2	3	4	5
Energy	1	2	3	4	5
Mental Clarity	1	2	3	4	5
Stress	1	2	3	4	5
Sleep Quality	1	2	3	4	5

Fasting Stability Journal

Daily Tracking Day _____

Day: ________________ Date: ________________

(5) Electrolytes / Fluids

Water ________________

Sodium ________________

Potassium ________________

Magnesium ________________

Caffeine ________________

Exercise / Sweating ________________

(6) Notes / Observations

(7) What Felt Stable?

(8) What Felt Unstable?

Fasting Stability Journal

Daily Tracking Day _____

Day: ____________________ Date: ____________________

1 Fasting Window

Start: ____________ End: ____________ Total Hours: ________

2 Eating Window

Start: ________________ End: ________________

3 Morning Stats

Weight ________________

Blood Glucose ________________

Ketones ________________

Blood Pressure ________________

Resting Heart Rate ________________

4 Daily Signals

Hunger	1	2	3	4	5
Cravings	1	2	3	4	5
Energy	1	2	3	4	5
Mental Clarity	1	2	3	4	5
Stress	1	2	3	4	5
Sleep Quality	1	2	3	4	5

Fasting Stability Journal

Daily Tracking Day _____

Day: ____________________ Date: ____________________

5 Electrolytes / Fluids

Water ____________________

Sodium ____________________

Potassium ____________________

Magnesium ____________________

Caffeine ____________________

Exercise / Sweating ____________________

6 Notes / Observations

____

____

____

____

____

____

7 What Felt Stable?

____

____

____

____

8 What Felt Unstable?

____

____

____

____

____

Fasting Stability Journal

Daily Tracking Day _____

Day: ____________________ Date: ____________________

1 Fasting Window

Start: ______________ End: ______________ Total Hours: __________

2 Eating Window

Start: ____________________ End: ______________

3 Morning Stats

Weight ____________________

Blood Glucose ______________

Ketones ____________________

Blood Pressure ______________

Resting Heart Rate ____________

4 Daily Signals

Hunger	1	2	3	4	5
Cravings	1	2	3	4	5
Energy	1	2	3	4	5
Mental Clarity	1	2	3	4	5
Stress	1	2	3	4	5
Sleep Quality	1	2	3	4	5

Fasting Stability Journal

Daily Tracking Day _____

Day: ____________________ Date: ____________________

⑤ Electrolytes / Fluids

Water ____________________

Sodium ____________________

Potassium ____________________

Magnesium ____________________

Caffeine ____________________

Exercise / Sweating ____________________

⑥ Notes / Observations

⑦ What Felt Stable?

⑧ What Felt Unstable?

Fasting Stability Journal

Weekly Review

① Cycle Review

Cycle Start: ____________ Cycle End: ____________ Days Tracked: ________

② Review Highlights

Most Stable Day: ______________________

Most Unstable Day: ______________________

Most Common Fasting Window: ______________________

Most Difficult Time of Day: ______________________

③ Signal Trends

Hunger	1	2	3	4	5
Cravings	1	2	3	4	5
Energy	1	2	3	4	5
Sleep	1	2	3	4	5
Stress	1	2	3	4	5

④ Main Patterns Noticed

____

____

____

____

⑤ What to Watch Next Cycle

____

____

____

____

____

Fasting Stability Journal

Daily Tracking Day _____

Day: ____________________ Date: ____________________

1 Fasting Window

Start: ______________ End: ______________ Total Hours: __________

2 Eating Window

Start: ____________________ End: ______________

3 Morning Stats

Weight ____________________

Blood Glucose ______________

Ketones ____________________

Blood Pressure ______________

Resting Heart Rate ___________

4 Daily Signals

Hunger	1	2	3	4	5
Cravings	1	2	3	4	5
Energy	1	2	3	4	5
Mental Clarity	1	2	3	4	5
Stress	1	2	3	4	5
Sleep Quality	1	2	3	4	5

Fasting Stability Journal

Daily Tracking Day _____

Day: ____________________ Date: ____________________

5 Electrolytes / Fluids

Water ____________________

Sodium ____________________

Potassium ____________________

Magnesium ____________________

Caffeine ____________________

Exercise / Sweating ____________________

6 Notes / Observations

7 What Felt Stable?

8 What Felt Unstable?

Fasting Stability Journal

Daily Tracking Day _____

Day: ____________________ Date: ____________________

① Fasting Window

Start: ____________ End: ____________ Total Hours: ________

② Eating Window

Start: ____________________ End: ________________

③ Morning Stats

Weight ____________________

Blood Glucose ________________

Ketones ____________________

Blood Pressure ________________

Resting Heart Rate ______________

④ Daily Signals

Hunger	1	2	3	4	5
Cravings	1	2	3	4	5
Energy	1	2	3	4	5
Mental Clarity	1	2	3	4	5
Stress	1	2	3	4	5
Sleep Quality	1	2	3	4	5

Fasting Stability Journal

Daily Tracking Day _____

Day: ____________________ Date: ____________________

5 Electrolytes / Fluids

Water ____________________

Sodium ____________________

Potassium ____________________

Magnesium ____________________

Caffeine ____________________

Exercise / Sweating ____________________

6 Notes / Observations

7 What Felt Stable?

8 What Felt Unstable?

Fasting Stability Journal

Daily Tracking Day _____

Day: ____________________ Date: ____________________

1 Fasting Window

Start: ______________ End: ______________ Total Hours: __________

2 Eating Window

Start: ____________________ End: ________________

3 Morning Stats

Weight ____________________

Blood Glucose ________________

Ketones ____________________

Blood Pressure ________________

Resting Heart Rate ______________

4 Daily Signals

Hunger	1	2	3	4	5
Cravings	1	2	3	4	5
Energy	1	2	3	4	5
Mental Clarity	1	2	3	4	5
Stress	1	2	3	4	5
Sleep Quality	1	2	3	4	5

Fasting Stability Journal

Daily Tracking Day _____

Day: ____________________ Date: ____________________

5 Electrolytes / Fluids

Water ____________________

Sodium ____________________

Potassium ____________________

Magnesium ____________________

Caffeine ____________________

Exercise / Sweating ____________________

6 Notes / Observations

7 What Felt Stable?

8 What Felt Unstable?

Fasting Stability Journal

Daily Tracking Day ____

Day: ____________________ Date: ____________________

1 Fasting Window

Start: ______________ End: ______________ Total Hours: ________

2 Eating Window

Start: ____________________ End: ______________

3 Morning Stats

Weight ____________________

Blood Glucose ______________

Ketones ____________________

Blood Pressure ______________

Resting Heart Rate ____________

4 Daily Signals

Hunger	1	2	3	4	5
Cravings	1	2	3	4	5
Energy	1	2	3	4	5
Mental Clarity	1	2	3	4	5
Stress	1	2	3	4	5
Sleep Quality	1	2	3	4	5

Fasting Stability Journal

Daily Tracking Day _____

Day: ____________________ Date: ____________________

(5) Electrolytes / Fluids

Water ____________________

Sodium ____________________

Potassium ____________________

Magnesium ____________________

Caffeine ____________________

Exercise / Sweating ____________________

(6) Notes / Observations

____

____

____

____

____

____

(7) What Felt Stable?

____

____

____

____

(8) What Felt Unstable?

____

____

____

____

____

Fasting Stability Journal

Daily Tracking Day _____

Day: ______________________ Date: ______________________

1 Fasting Window

Start: ______________ End: ______________ Total Hours: __________

2 Eating Window

Start: ______________________ End: ______________________

3 Morning Stats

Weight ______________________

Blood Glucose ______________________

Ketones ______________________

Blood Pressure ______________________

Resting Heart Rate ______________________

4 Daily Signals

Hunger	1	2	3	4	5
Cravings	1	2	3	4	5
Energy	1	2	3	4	5
Mental Clarity	1	2	3	4	5
Stress	1	2	3	4	5
Sleep Quality	1	2	3	4	5

Fasting Stability Journal

Daily Tracking Day _____

Day: ____________________ Date: ____________________

5 Electrolytes / Fluids

Water ____________________

Sodium ____________________

Potassium ____________________

Magnesium ____________________

Caffeine ____________________

Exercise / Sweating ____________________

6 Notes / Observations

7 What Felt Stable?

8 What Felt Unstable?

Fasting Stability Journal

Daily Tracking Day _____

Day: ____________________ Date: ____________________

1 Fasting Window

Start: ______________ End: ____________ Total Hours: ________

2 Eating Window

Start: ____________________ End: ________________

3 Morning Stats

Weight ____________________

Blood Glucose ________________

Ketones ____________________

Blood Pressure ________________

Resting Heart Rate ______________

4 Daily Signals

Hunger	1	2	3	4	5
Cravings	1	2	3	4	5
Energy	1	2	3	4	5
Mental Clarity	1	2	3	4	5
Stress	1	2	3	4	5
Sleep Quality	1	2	3	4	5

Fasting Stability Journal

Daily Tracking Day _____

Day: ____________________ Date: ____________________

⑤ Electrolytes / Fluids

Water ____________________

Sodium ____________________

Potassium ____________________

Magnesium ____________________

Caffeine ____________________

Exercise / Sweating ____________________

⑥ Notes / Observations

⑦ What Felt Stable?

⑧ What Felt Unstable?

Fasting Stability Journal

Daily Tracking Day ____

Day: ____________________ Date: ____________________

1 Fasting Window

Start: ______________ End: ______________ Total Hours: __________

2 Eating Window

Start: ____________________ End: ____________________

3 Morning Stats

Weight ____________________

Blood Glucose ________________

Ketones ____________________

Blood Pressure ________________

Resting Heart Rate ______________

4 Daily Signals

Hunger	1	2	3	4	5
Cravings	1	2	3	4	5
Energy	1	2	3	4	5
Mental Clarity	1	2	3	4	5
Stress	1	2	3	4	5
Sleep Quality	1	2	3	4	5

Fasting Stability Journal

Daily Tracking Day _____

Day: ____________________ Date: ____________________

5 Electrolytes / Fluids

Water ____________________

Sodium ____________________

Potassium ____________________

Magnesium ____________________

Caffeine ____________________

Exercise / Sweating ____________________

6 Notes / Observations

7 What Felt Stable?

8 What Felt Unstable?

Fasting Stability Journal

Weekly Review

1 Cycle Review

Cycle Start: ____________ Cycle End: ____________ Days Tracked: ________

2 Review Highlights

Most Stable Day: ____________________

Most Unstable Day: ____________________

Most Common Fasting Window: ____________________

Most Difficult Time of Day: ____________________

3 Signal Trends

Hunger	1	2	3	4	5
Cravings	1	2	3	4	5
Energy	1	2	3	4	5
Sleep	1	2	3	4	5
Stress	1	2	3	4	5

4 Main Patterns Noticed

____

____

____

____

5 What to Watch Next Cycle

____

____

____

____

____

Fasting Stability Journal

Daily Tracking Day _____

Day: ____________________ Date: ____________________

1 Fasting Window

Start: ______________ End: ______________ Total Hours: __________

2 Eating Window

Start: ____________________ End: ____________________

3 Morning Stats

Weight ____________________

Blood Glucose ____________________

Ketones ____________________

Blood Pressure ____________________

Resting Heart Rate ____________________

4 Daily Signals

Hunger	1	2	3	4	5
Cravings	1	2	3	4	5
Energy	1	2	3	4	5
Mental Clarity	1	2	3	4	5
Stress	1	2	3	4	5
Sleep Quality	1	2	3	4	5

Fasting Stability Journal

Daily Tracking Day _____

Day: ____________________ Date: ____________________

(5) Electrolytes / Fluids

Water ____________________

Sodium ____________________

Potassium ____________________

Magnesium ____________________

Caffeine ____________________

Exercise / Sweating ____________________

(6) Notes / Observations

(7) What Felt Stable?

(8) What Felt Unstable?

Fasting Stability Journal

Daily Tracking Day _____

Day: ______________________ Date: ______________________

1 Fasting Window

Start: ______________ End: ______________ Total Hours: __________

2 Eating Window

Start: ______________________ End: ______________________

3 Morning Stats

Weight ______________________

Blood Glucose ______________________

Ketones ______________________

Blood Pressure ______________________

Resting Heart Rate ______________________

4 Daily Signals

Hunger	1	2	3	4	5
Cravings	1	2	3	4	5
Energy	1	2	3	4	5
Mental Clarity	1	2	3	4	5
Stress	1	2	3	4	5
Sleep Quality	1	2	3	4	5

Fasting Stability Journal

Daily Tracking Day _____

Day: ____________________ Date: ____________________

(5) Electrolytes / Fluids

Water ____________________

Sodium ____________________

Potassium ____________________

Magnesium ____________________

Caffeine ____________________

Exercise / Sweating ____________________

(6) Notes / Observations

____

____

____

____

____

____

(7) What Felt Stable?

____

____

____

____

(8) What Felt Unstable?

____

____

____

____

____

Fasting Stability Journal

Daily Tracking Day _____

Day: ______________________ Date: ______________________

1 Fasting Window

Start: ______________ End: ______________ Total Hours: __________

2 Eating Window

Start: ____________________ End: ________________

3 Morning Stats

Weight ____________________

Blood Glucose ________________

Ketones ____________________

Blood Pressure ________________

Resting Heart Rate ______________

4 Daily Signals

Hunger	1	2	3	4	5
Cravings	1	2	3	4	5
Energy	1	2	3	4	5
Mental Clarity	1	2	3	4	5
Stress	1	2	3	4	5
Sleep Quality	1	2	3	4	5

Fasting Stability Journal

Daily Tracking Day _____

Day: ________________ Date: ________________

(5) Electrolytes / Fluids

Water ____________________

Sodium ____________________

Potassium ____________________

Magnesium ____________________

Caffeine ____________________

Exercise / Sweating ____________________

(6) Notes / Observations

(7) What Felt Stable?

(8) What Felt Unstable?

Fasting Stability Journal

Daily Tracking Day _____

Day: ______________________ Date: ______________________

1 Fasting Window

Start: ______________ End: ______________ Total Hours: __________

2 Eating Window

Start: ______________________ End: ______________________

3 Morning Stats

Weight ______________________

Blood Glucose ______________________

Ketones ______________________

Blood Pressure ______________________

Resting Heart Rate ______________________

4 Daily Signals

Hunger	1	2	3	4	5
Cravings	1	2	3	4	5
Energy	1	2	3	4	5
Mental Clarity	1	2	3	4	5
Stress	1	2	3	4	5
Sleep Quality	1	2	3	4	5

Fasting Stability Journal

Daily Tracking Day _____

Day: ____________________ Date: ____________________

5 Electrolytes / Fluids

Water ____________________

Sodium ____________________

Potassium ____________________

Magnesium ____________________

Caffeine ____________________

Exercise / Sweating ____________________

6 Notes / Observations

7 What Felt Stable?

8 What Felt Unstable?

Fasting Stability Journal

Daily Tracking Day _____

Day: ____________________ Date: ____________________

1 Fasting Window

Start: ______________ End: ______________ Total Hours: __________

2 Eating Window

Start: ____________________ End: ______________

3 Morning Stats

Weight ____________________

Blood Glucose ______________

Ketones ____________________

Blood Pressure ______________

Resting Heart Rate ______________

4 Daily Signals

Hunger	1	2	3	4	5
Cravings	1	2	3	4	5
Energy	1	2	3	4	5
Mental Clarity	1	2	3	4	5
Stress	1	2	3	4	5
Sleep Quality	1	2	3	4	5

Fasting Stability Journal

Daily Tracking Day _____

Day: ____________________ Date: ____________________

(5) Electrolytes / Fluids

Water ____________________

Sodium ____________________

Potassium ____________________

Magnesium ____________________

Caffeine ____________________

Exercise / Sweating ____________________

(6) Notes / Observations

____

____

____

____

____

____

(7) What Felt Stable?

____

____

____

____

(8) What Felt Unstable?

____

____

____

____

____

Fasting Stability Journal

Daily Tracking Day ____

Day: ______________________ Date: ______________________

1 Fasting Window

Start: ____________ End: ____________ Total Hours: ________

2 Eating Window

Start: ________________ End: ______________

3 Morning Stats

Weight ________________

Blood Glucose ______________

Ketones ________________

Blood Pressure ______________

Resting Heart Rate ____________

4 Daily Signals

Hunger	1	2	3	4	5
Cravings	1	2	3	4	5
Energy	1	2	3	4	5
Mental Clarity	1	2	3	4	5
Stress	1	2	3	4	5
Sleep Quality	1	2	3	4	5

Fasting Stability Journal

Daily Tracking Day ____

Day: ______________ Date: ______________

5 Electrolytes / Fluids

Water ______________

Sodium ______________

Potassium ______________

Magnesium ______________

Caffeine ______________

Exercise / Sweating ______________

6 Notes / Observations

7 What Felt Stable?

8 What Felt Unstable?

Fasting Stability Journal

Daily Tracking Day _____

Day: ______________________ Date: ______________________

1 Fasting Window

Start: ______________ End: ______________ Total Hours: __________

2 Eating Window

Start: ______________________ End: ______________________

3 Morning Stats

Weight ______________________

Blood Glucose ______________________

Ketones ______________________

Blood Pressure ______________________

Resting Heart Rate ______________________

4 Daily Signals

Hunger	1	2	3	4	5
Cravings	1	2	3	4	5
Energy	1	2	3	4	5
Mental Clarity	1	2	3	4	5
Stress	1	2	3	4	5
Sleep Quality	1	2	3	4	5

Fasting Stability Journal

Daily Tracking Day _____

Day: ____________________ Date: ____________________

(5) Electrolytes / Fluids

Water ____________________

Sodium ____________________

Potassium ____________________

Magnesium ____________________

Caffeine ____________________

Exercise / Sweating ____________________

(6) Notes / Observations

(7) What Felt Stable?

(8) What Felt Unstable?

Fasting Stability Journal

Weekly Review

① Cycle Review

Cycle Start: ________________ Cycle End: ______________ Days Tracked: ________

② Review Highlights

Most Stable Day: ____

Most Unstable Day: ____

Most Common Fasting Window: ______________________________________

Most Difficult Time of Day: ____

③ Signal Trends

Hunger	1	2	3	4	5
Cravings	1	2	3	4	5
Energy	1	2	3	4	5
Sleep	1	2	3	4	5
Stress	1	2	3	4	5

④ Main Patterns Noticed

____

____

____

____

⑤ What to Watch Next Cycle

____

____

____

____

____

Fasting Stability Journal

Daily Tracking Day _____

Day: ______________________ Date: ______________________

1 Fasting Window

Start: ______________ End: ______________ Total Hours: __________

2 Eating Window

Start: ______________________ End: ______________________

3 Morning Stats

Weight ______________________

Blood Glucose ______________________

Ketones ______________________

Blood Pressure ______________________

Resting Heart Rate ______________________

4 Daily Signals

Hunger	1	2	3	4	5
Cravings	1	2	3	4	5
Energy	1	2	3	4	5
Mental Clarity	1	2	3	4	5
Stress	1	2	3	4	5
Sleep Quality	1	2	3	4	5

Fasting Stability Journal

Daily Tracking Day _____

Day: ____________________ Date: ____________________

(5) Electrolytes / Fluids

Water ____________________

Sodium ____________________

Potassium ____________________

Magnesium ____________________

Caffeine ____________________

Exercise / Sweating ____________________

(6) Notes / Observations

____

____

____

____

____

____

(7) What Felt Stable?

____

____

____

____

(8) What Felt Unstable?

____

____

____

____

____

Fasting Stability Journal

Daily Tracking Day ____

Day: ______________________ Date: ______________________

1 Fasting Window

Start: ______________ End: ______________ Total Hours: ________

2 Eating Window

Start: ______________________ End: ________________

3 Morning Stats

Weight ______________________

Blood Glucose ________________

Ketones ______________________

Blood Pressure ________________

Resting Heart Rate ______________

4 Daily Signals

Hunger	1	2	3	4	5
Cravings	1	2	3	4	5
Energy	1	2	3	4	5
Mental Clarity	1	2	3	4	5
Stress	1	2	3	4	5
Sleep Quality	1	2	3	4	5

Fasting Stability Journal

Daily Tracking Day _____

Day: ________________ Date: ________________

5 Electrolytes / Fluids

Water ________________

Sodium ________________

Potassium ________________

Magnesium ________________

Caffeine ________________

Exercise / Sweating ________________

6 Notes / Observations

7 What Felt Stable?

8 What Felt Unstable?

Fasting Stability Journal

Daily Tracking Day _____

Day: ____________________ Date: ____________________

1 Fasting Window

Start: ______________ End: ______________ Total Hours: __________

2 Eating Window

Start: ____________________ End: ____________________

3 Morning Stats

Weight ____________________

Blood Glucose ____________________

Ketones ____________________

Blood Pressure ____________________

Resting Heart Rate ____________________

4 Daily Signals

Hunger	1	2	3	4	5
Cravings	1	2	3	4	5
Energy	1	2	3	4	5
Mental Clarity	1	2	3	4	5
Stress	1	2	3	4	5
Sleep Quality	1	2	3	4	5

Fasting Stability Journal

Daily Tracking Day _____

Day: ____________________ Date: ____________________

(5) Electrolytes / Fluids

Water ____________________

Sodium ____________________

Potassium ____________________

Magnesium ____________________

Caffeine ____________________

Exercise / Sweating ____________________

(6) Notes / Observations

(7) What Felt Stable?

(8) What Felt Unstable?

Fasting Stability Journal

Daily Tracking Day _____

Day: ______________________ Date: ______________________

1 Fasting Window

Start: ______________ End: ______________ Total Hours: __________

2 Eating Window

Start: ______________________ End: __________________

3 Morning Stats

Weight ______________________

Blood Glucose ______________________

Ketones ______________________

Blood Pressure ______________________

Resting Heart Rate ______________________

4 Daily Signals

Hunger	1	2	3	4	5
Cravings	1	2	3	4	5
Energy	1	2	3	4	5
Mental Clarity	1	2	3	4	5
Stress	1	2	3	4	5
Sleep Quality	1	2	3	4	5

Fasting Stability Journal

Daily Tracking Day _____

Day: ____________________ Date: ____________________

(5) Electrolytes / Fluids

Water ____________________

Sodium ____________________

Potassium ____________________

Magnesium ____________________

Caffeine ____________________

Exercise / Sweating ____________________

(6) Notes / Observations

____

____

____

____

____

____

(7) What Felt Stable?

____

____

____

____

(8) What Felt Unstable?

____

____

____

____

____

Fasting Stability Journal

Daily Tracking Day _____

Day: ______________________ Date: ______________________

1 Fasting Window

Start: ______________ End: ______________ Total Hours: __________

2 Eating Window

Start: ______________________ End: __________________

3 Morning Stats

Weight ____________________

Blood Glucose ____________________

Ketones ____________________

Blood Pressure ____________________

Resting Heart Rate ____________________

4 Daily Signals

Hunger	1	2	3	4	5
Cravings	1	2	3	4	5
Energy	1	2	3	4	5
Mental Clarity	1	2	3	4	5
Stress	1	2	3	4	5
Sleep Quality	1	2	3	4	5

Fasting Stability Journal

Daily Tracking Day _____

Day: ________________ Date: ________________

(5) Electrolytes / Fluids

Water ______________________________

Sodium ______________________________

Potassium ______________________________

Magnesium ______________________________

Caffeine ______________________________

Exercise / Sweating ______________________________

(6) Notes / Observations

____

____

____

____

____

____

(7) What Felt Stable?

____

____

____

____

(8) What Felt Unstable?

____

____

____

____

____

Fasting Stability Journal

Daily Tracking Day ____

Day: ____________________ Date: ____________________

1 Fasting Window

Start: ______________ End: ______________ Total Hours: __________

2 Eating Window

Start: ____________________ End: ____________________

3 Morning Stats

Weight ____________________

Blood Glucose ____________________

Ketones ____________________

Blood Pressure ____________________

Resting Heart Rate ____________________

4 Daily Signals

Hunger	1	2	3	4	5
Cravings	1	2	3	4	5
Energy	1	2	3	4	5
Mental Clarity	1	2	3	4	5
Stress	1	2	3	4	5
Sleep Quality	1	2	3	4	5

Fasting Stability Journal

Daily Tracking Day _____

Day: ____________________ Date: ____________________

5 Electrolytes / Fluids

Water ____________________

Sodium ____________________

Potassium ____________________

Magnesium ____________________

Caffeine ____________________

Exercise / Sweating ____________________

6 Notes / Observations

7 What Felt Stable?

8 What Felt Unstable?

Fasting Stability Journal

Daily Tracking Day _____

Day: ____________________ Date: ____________________

1 Fasting Window

Start: ______________ End: ______________ Total Hours: __________

2 Eating Window

Start: ____________________ End: ______________

3 Morning Stats

Weight ____________________

Blood Glucose ________________

Ketones ____________________

Blood Pressure ________________

Resting Heart Rate ______________

4 Daily Signals

Hunger	1	2	3	4	5
Cravings	1	2	3	4	5
Energy	1	2	3	4	5
Mental Clarity	1	2	3	4	5
Stress	1	2	3	4	5
Sleep Quality	1	2	3	4	5

Fasting Stability Journal

Daily Tracking Day _____

Day: ____________________ Date: ____________________

⑤ Electrolytes / Fluids

Water ____________________

Sodium ____________________

Potassium ____________________

Magnesium ____________________

Caffeine ____________________

Exercise / Sweating ____________________

⑥ Notes / Observations

⑦ What Felt Stable?

⑧ What Felt Unstable?

Fasting Stability Journal

Weekly Review

① Cycle Review

Cycle Start: ____________ Cycle End: ____________ Days Tracked: ________

② Review Highlights

Most Stable Day: ____________

Most Unstable Day: ____________

Most Common Fasting Window: ____________

Most Difficult Time of Day: ____________

③ Signal Trends

Hunger	1	2	3	4	5
Cravings	1	2	3	4	5
Energy	1	2	3	4	5
Sleep	1	2	3	4	5
Stress	1	2	3	4	5

④ Main Patterns Noticed

____

____

____

____

⑤ What to Watch Next Cycle

____

____

____

____

____

Fasting Stability Journal

Daily Tracking Day _____

Day: ______________________ Date: ______________________

1 Fasting Window

Start: ______________ End: ______________ Total Hours: __________

2 Eating Window

Start: ______________________ End: ______________________

3 Morning Stats

Weight ______________________

Blood Glucose ______________________

Ketones ______________________

Blood Pressure ______________________

Resting Heart Rate ______________________

4 Daily Signals

Hunger	1	2	3	4	5
Cravings	1	2	3	4	5
Energy	1	2	3	4	5
Mental Clarity	1	2	3	4	5
Stress	1	2	3	4	5
Sleep Quality	1	2	3	4	5

Fasting Stability Journal

Daily Tracking Day _____

Day: ____________________ Date: ____________________

5 Electrolytes / Fluids

Water ____________________

Sodium ____________________

Potassium ____________________

Magnesium ____________________

Caffeine ____________________

Exercise / Sweating ____________________

6 Notes / Observations

____

____

____

____

____

____

7 What Felt Stable?

____

____

____

____

8 What Felt Unstable?

____

____

____

____

____

Fasting Stability Journal

Daily Tracking Day _____

Day: ______________________ Date: ______________________

1 Fasting Window

Start: ______________ End: ______________ Total Hours: __________

2 Eating Window

Start: ____________________ End: ________________

3 Morning Stats

Weight ____________________

Blood Glucose ________________

Ketones ____________________

Blood Pressure ________________

Resting Heart Rate ______________

4 Daily Signals

Hunger	1	2	3	4	5
Cravings	1	2	3	4	5
Energy	1	2	3	4	5
Mental Clarity	1	2	3	4	5
Stress	1	2	3	4	5
Sleep Quality	1	2	3	4	5

Fasting Stability Journal

Daily Tracking Day _____

Day: ____________________ Date: ____________________

(5) Electrolytes / Fluids

Water ____________________

Sodium ____________________

Potassium ____________________

Magnesium ____________________

Caffeine ____________________

Exercise / Sweating ____________________

(6) Notes / Observations

____

____

____

____

____

____

(7) What Felt Stable?

____

____

____

____

(8) What Felt Unstable?

____

____

____

____

____

Fasting Stability Journal

Daily Tracking Day _____

Day: ____________________ Date: ____________________

1 Fasting Window

Start: ______________ End: ______________ Total Hours: __________

2 Eating Window

Start: ____________________ End: ______________

3 Morning Stats

Weight ______________

Blood Glucose ______________

Ketones ______________

Blood Pressure ______________

Resting Heart Rate ______________

4 Daily Signals

Hunger	1	2	3	4	5
Cravings	1	2	3	4	5
Energy	1	2	3	4	5
Mental Clarity	1	2	3	4	5
Stress	1	2	3	4	5
Sleep Quality	1	2	3	4	5

Fasting Stability Journal

Daily Tracking Day _____

Day: ____________________ Date: ____________________

(5) Electrolytes / Fluids

Water ______________________________

Sodium ______________________________

Potassium ______________________________

Magnesium ______________________________

Caffeine ______________________________

Exercise / Sweating ______________________________

(6) Notes / Observations

____

____

____

____

____

____

(7) What Felt Stable?

____

____

____

____

(8) What Felt Unstable?

____

____

____

____

____

Fasting Stability Journal

Daily Tracking Day ____

Day: ______________________ Date: ______________________

1 Fasting Window

Start: ______________ End: ______________ Total Hours: __________

2 Eating Window

Start: ______________________ End: ____________________

3 Morning Stats

Weight ____________________

Blood Glucose ____________________

Ketones ____________________

Blood Pressure ____________________

Resting Heart Rate ____________________

4 Daily Signals

Hunger	1	2	3	4	5
Cravings	1	2	3	4	5
Energy	1	2	3	4	5
Mental Clarity	1	2	3	4	5
Stress	1	2	3	4	5
Sleep Quality	1	2	3	4	5

Fasting Stability Journal

Daily Tracking Day _____

Day: ____________________ Date: ____________________

(5) Electrolytes / Fluids

Water ____________________

Sodium ____________________

Potassium ____________________

Magnesium ____________________

Caffeine ____________________

Exercise / Sweating ____________________

(6) Notes / Observations

(7) What Felt Stable?

(8) What Felt Unstable?

Fasting Stability Journal

Daily Tracking Day ____

Day: ______________________ Date: ______________________

1 Fasting Window

Start: ______________ End: ______________ Total Hours: __________

2 Eating Window

Start: ______________________ End: ______________________

3 Morning Stats

Weight ______________________

Blood Glucose ______________________

Ketones ______________________

Blood Pressure ______________________

Resting Heart Rate ______________________

4 Daily Signals

Hunger	1	2	3	4	5
Cravings	1	2	3	4	5
Energy	1	2	3	4	5
Mental Clarity	1	2	3	4	5
Stress	1	2	3	4	5
Sleep Quality	1	2	3	4	5

Fasting Stability Journal

Daily Tracking Day _____

Day: ____________________ Date: ____________________

5 Electrolytes / Fluids

Water ____________________

Sodium ____________________

Potassium ____________________

Magnesium ____________________

Caffeine ____________________

Exercise / Sweating ____________________

6 Notes / Observations

7 What Felt Stable?

8 What Felt Unstable?

Fasting Stability Journal

Daily Tracking Day _____

Day: ______________________ Date: ______________________

1 Fasting Window

Start: ______________ End: ______________ Total Hours: __________

2 Eating Window

Start: ______________ End: ______________

3 Morning Stats

Weight ______________

Blood Glucose ______________

Ketones ______________

Blood Pressure ______________

Resting Heart Rate ______________

4 Daily Signals

Hunger	1	2	3	4	5
Cravings	1	2	3	4	5
Energy	1	2	3	4	5
Mental Clarity	1	2	3	4	5
Stress	1	2	3	4	5
Sleep Quality	1	2	3	4	5

Fasting Stability Journal

Daily Tracking Day _____

Day: ____________________ Date: ____________________

5 Electrolytes / Fluids

Water ____________________

Sodium ____________________

Potassium ____________________

Magnesium ____________________

Caffeine ____________________

Exercise / Sweating ____________________

6 Notes / Observations

7 What Felt Stable?

8 What Felt Unstable?

Fasting Stability Journal

Daily Tracking Day ____

Day: ______________________ Date: ______________________

1 Fasting Window

Start: ______________ End: ______________ Total Hours: __________

2 Eating Window

Start: ______________________ End: ______________________

3 Morning Stats

Weight ______________________

Blood Glucose ______________________

Ketones ______________________

Blood Pressure ______________________

Resting Heart Rate ______________________

4 Daily Signals

Hunger	1	2	3	4	5
Cravings	1	2	3	4	5
Energy	1	2	3	4	5
Mental Clarity	1	2	3	4	5
Stress	1	2	3	4	5
Sleep Quality	1	2	3	4	5

Fasting Stability Journal

Daily Tracking Day _____

Day: ____________________ Date: ____________________

5 Electrolytes / Fluids

Water ____________________

Sodium ____________________

Potassium ____________________

Magnesium ____________________

Caffeine ____________________

Exercise / Sweating ____________________

6 Notes / Observations

7 What Felt Stable?

8 What Felt Unstable?

6-WEEK REVIEW

Weeks __________ to __________ Date ________________

1. OVERALL PROGRESS

How would I describe my progress over this 6-week period?

____

____

____

____

____

2. BIGGEST WINS

What are my top 3 wins?

1. ______________________________
   ____
   ____
2. ______________________________
   ____
   ____
3. ______________________________
   ____
   ____

2. BIGGEST CHALLENGES

What were my biggest challenges?

1. ______________________________
   ____
   ____
2. ______________________________
   ____
   ____
3. ______________________________
   ____
   ____

3. WHAT I'VE LEARNED

Key lessons from this 6-week period.

____

____

____

____

4. NEXT 6 WEEKS FOCUS

What I will focus on next.

____

____

____

____

____

Fasting Stability Journal

Daily Tracking Day _____

Day: ______________________ Date: ______________________

1 Fasting Window

Start: ______________ End: ______________ Total Hours: __________

2 Eating Window

Start: ______________________ End: ______________________

3 Morning Stats

Weight ______________________

Blood Glucose ______________________

Ketones ______________________

Blood Pressure ______________________

Resting Heart Rate ______________________

4 Daily Signals

Hunger	1	2	3	4	5
Cravings	1	2	3	4	5
Energy	1	2	3	4	5
Mental Clarity	1	2	3	4	5
Stress	1	2	3	4	5
Sleep Quality	1	2	3	4	5

Fasting Stability Journal

Daily Tracking Day _____

Day: ____________________ Date: ____________________

5 Electrolytes / Fluids

Water ____________________

Sodium ____________________

Potassium ____________________

Magnesium ____________________

Caffeine ____________________

Exercise / Sweating ____________________

6 Notes / Observations

7 What Felt Stable?

8 What Felt Unstable?

Fasting Stability Journal

Daily Tracking Day ____

Day: ______________________ Date: ______________________

1 Fasting Window

Start: ______________ End: ______________ Total Hours: __________

2 Eating Window

Start: ______________________ End: ______________________

3 Morning Stats

Weight ______________________

Blood Glucose ______________________

Ketones ______________________

Blood Pressure ______________________

Resting Heart Rate ______________________

4 Daily Signals

Hunger	1	2	3	4	5
Cravings	1	2	3	4	5
Energy	1	2	3	4	5
Mental Clarity	1	2	3	4	5
Stress	1	2	3	4	5
Sleep Quality	1	2	3	4	5

Fasting Stability Journal

Daily Tracking Day _____

Day: ____________________ Date: ____________________

⑤ Electrolytes / Fluids

Water ____________________

Sodium ____________________

Potassium ____________________

Magnesium ____________________

Caffeine ____________________

Exercise / Sweating ____________________

⑥ Notes / Observations

____

____

____

____

____

____

⑦ What Felt Stable?

____

____

____

____

⑧ What Felt Unstable?

____

____

____

____

____

Fasting Stability Journal

Daily Tracking Day _____

Day: ____________________ Date: ____________________

1 Fasting Window

Start: ______________ End: ______________ Total Hours: __________

2 Eating Window

Start: ____________________ End: ______________

3 Morning Stats

Weight ____________________

Blood Glucose ________________

Ketones ____________________

Blood Pressure ________________

Resting Heart Rate ______________

4 Daily Signals

Hunger	1	2	3	4	5
Cravings	1	2	3	4	5
Energy	1	2	3	4	5
Mental Clarity	1	2	3	4	5
Stress	1	2	3	4	5
Sleep Quality	1	2	3	4	5

Fasting Stability Journal

Daily Tracking Day _____

Day: ____________________ Date: ____________________

(5) Electrolytes / Fluids

Water ____________________

Sodium ____________________

Potassium ____________________

Magnesium ____________________

Caffeine ____________________

Exercise / Sweating ____________________

(6) Notes / Observations

____

____

____

____

____

____

(7) What Felt Stable?

____

____

____

____

(8) What Felt Unstable?

____

____

____

____

____

Fasting Stability Journal

Daily Tracking Day _____

Day: ____________________ Date: ____________________

1 Fasting Window

Start: ______________ End: ______________ Total Hours: __________

2 Eating Window

Start: ____________________ End: ______________

3 Morning Stats

Weight ____________________

Blood Glucose ______________

Ketones ____________________

Blood Pressure ______________

Resting Heart Rate ____________

4 Daily Signals

Hunger	1	2	3	4	5
Cravings	1	2	3	4	5
Energy	1	2	3	4	5
Mental Clarity	1	2	3	4	5
Stress	1	2	3	4	5
Sleep Quality	1	2	3	4	5

Fasting Stability Journal

Daily Tracking Day _____

Day: ____________________ Date: ____________________

(5) Electrolytes / Fluids

Water ____________________

Sodium ____________________

Potassium ____________________

Magnesium ____________________

Caffeine ____________________

Exercise / Sweating ____________________

(6) Notes / Observations

(7) What Felt Stable?

(8) What Felt Unstable?

Fasting Stability Journal

Daily Tracking Day ____

Day: ______________________ **Date:** ______________________

① Fasting Window

Start: ______________ End: ______________ Total Hours: __________

② Eating Window

Start: ______________________ End: ______________________

③ Morning Stats

Weight ______________________

Blood Glucose ______________________

Ketones ______________________

Blood Pressure ______________________

Resting Heart Rate ______________________

④ Daily Signals

Hunger	1	2	3	4	5
Cravings	1	2	3	4	5
Energy	1	2	3	4	5
Mental Clarity	1	2	3	4	5
Stress	1	2	3	4	5
Sleep Quality	1	2	3	4	5

Fasting Stability Journal

Daily Tracking Day _____

Day: ________________ Date: ________________

(5) Electrolytes / Fluids

Water ________________

Sodium ________________

Potassium ________________

Magnesium ________________

Caffeine ________________

Exercise / Sweating ________________

(6) Notes / Observations

____

____

____

____

____

____

(7) What Felt Stable?

____

____

____

____

(8) What Felt Unstable?

____

____

____

____

____

Fasting Stability Journal

Daily Tracking Day _____

Day: ____________________ Date: ____________________

1 Fasting Window

Start: ______________ End: ______________ Total Hours: __________

2 Eating Window

Start: ____________________ End: ____________________

3 Morning Stats

Weight ____________________

Blood Glucose ____________________

Ketones ____________________

Blood Pressure ____________________

Resting Heart Rate ____________________

4 Daily Signals

Hunger	1	2	3	4	5
Cravings	1	2	3	4	5
Energy	1	2	3	4	5
Mental Clarity	1	2	3	4	5
Stress	1	2	3	4	5
Sleep Quality	1	2	3	4	5

Fasting Stability Journal

Daily Tracking Day _____

Day: ____________________ Date: ____________________

5 Electrolytes / Fluids

Water ____________________

Sodium ____________________

Potassium ____________________

Magnesium ____________________

Caffeine ____________________

Exercise / Sweating ____________________

6 Notes / Observations

____

____

____

____

____

____

7 What Felt Stable?

____

____

____

____

8 What Felt Unstable?

____

____

____

____

____

Fasting Stability Journal

Daily Tracking Day ____

Day: ____________________ Date: ____________________

1 Fasting Window

Start: ____________ End: ____________ Total Hours: ________

2 Eating Window

Start: ________________ End: ______________

3 Morning Stats

Weight ________________

Blood Glucose ________________

Ketones ________________

Blood Pressure ________________

Resting Heart Rate ________________

4 Daily Signals

Hunger	1	2	3	4	5
Cravings	1	2	3	4	5
Energy	1	2	3	4	5
Mental Clarity	1	2	3	4	5
Stress	1	2	3	4	5
Sleep Quality	1	2	3	4	5

Fasting Stability Journal

Daily Tracking Day _____

Day: ____________________ Date: ____________________

(5) Electrolytes / Fluids

Water ____________________

Sodium ____________________

Potassium ____________________

Magnesium ____________________

Caffeine ____________________

Exercise / Sweating ____________________

(6) Notes / Observations

(7) What Felt Stable?

(8) What Felt Unstable?

Fasting Stability Journal

Weekly Review

1 Cycle Review

Cycle Start: ____________ Cycle End: ____________ Days Tracked: ________

2 Review Highlights

Most Stable Day: ____________________

Most Unstable Day: ____________________

Most Common Fasting Window: ____________________

Most Difficult Time of Day: ____________________

3 Signal Trends

Hunger	1	2	3	4	5
Cravings	1	2	3	4	5
Energy	1	2	3	4	5
Sleep	1	2	3	4	5
Stress	1	2	3	4	5

4 Main Patterns Noticed

____

____

____

____

5 What to Watch Next Cycle

____

____

____

____

____

Fasting Stability Journal

Daily Tracking Day _____

Day: ____________________ Date: ____________________

1 Fasting Window

Start: ______________ End: ______________ Total Hours: __________

2 Eating Window

Start: ____________________ End: ________________

3 Morning Stats

Weight ____________________

Blood Glucose ________________

Ketones ____________________

Blood Pressure ________________

Resting Heart Rate ______________

4 Daily Signals

Hunger	1	2	3	4	5
Cravings	1	2	3	4	5
Energy	1	2	3	4	5
Mental Clarity	1	2	3	4	5
Stress	1	2	3	4	5
Sleep Quality	1	2	3	4	5

Fasting Stability Journal

Daily Tracking Day _____

Day: ____________________ Date: ____________________

5 Electrolytes / Fluids

Water ____________________

Sodium ____________________

Potassium ____________________

Magnesium ____________________

Caffeine ____________________

Exercise / Sweating ____________________

6 Notes / Observations

7 What Felt Stable?

8 What Felt Unstable?

Fasting Stability Journal

Daily Tracking Day _____

Day: ______________________ Date: ______________________

(1) Fasting Window

Start: ______________ End: ______________ Total Hours: __________

(2) Eating Window

Start: ______________ End: ______________

(3) Morning Stats

Weight ______________

Blood Glucose ______________

Ketones ______________

Blood Pressure ______________

Resting Heart Rate ______________

(4) Daily Signals

Hunger	1	2	3	4	5
Cravings	1	2	3	4	5
Energy	1	2	3	4	5
Mental Clarity	1	2	3	4	5
Stress	1	2	3	4	5
Sleep Quality	1	2	3	4	5

Fasting Stability Journal

Daily Tracking Day _____

Day: ____________________ Date: ____________________

(5) Electrolytes / Fluids

Water ______________________________

Sodium ______________________________

Potassium ______________________________

Magnesium ______________________________

Caffeine ______________________________

Exercise / Sweating ______________________________

(6) Notes / Observations

____

____

____

____

____

____

(7) What Felt Stable?

____

____

____

____

(8) What Felt Unstable?

____

____

____

____

____

Fasting Stability Journal

Daily Tracking Day ____

Day: ______________________ Date: ______________________

1 Fasting Window

Start: ______________ End: ______________ Total Hours: __________

2 Eating Window

Start: ______________________ End: ______________________

3 Morning Stats

Weight ______________________

Blood Glucose ______________________

Ketones ______________________

Blood Pressure ______________________

Resting Heart Rate ______________________

4 Daily Signals

Hunger	1	2	3	4	5
Cravings	1	2	3	4	5
Energy	1	2	3	4	5
Mental Clarity	1	2	3	4	5
Stress	1	2	3	4	5
Sleep Quality	1	2	3	4	5

Fasting Stability Journal

Daily Tracking Day _____

Day: ____________________ Date: ____________________

5 Electrolytes / Fluids

Water ____________________

Sodium ____________________

Potassium ____________________

Magnesium ____________________

Caffeine ____________________

Exercise / Sweating ____________________

6 Notes / Observations

____

____

____

____

____

____

7 What Felt Stable?

____

____

____

____

8 What Felt Unstable?

____

____

____

____

____

Fasting Stability Journal

Daily Tracking Day ____

Day: ______________________ Date: ______________________

1 Fasting Window

Start: ______________ End: ______________ Total Hours: __________

2 Eating Window

Start: ______________________ End: ______________________

3 Morning Stats

Weight ______________________

Blood Glucose ______________________

Ketones ______________________

Blood Pressure ______________________

Resting Heart Rate ______________________

4 Daily Signals

Hunger	1	2	3	4	5
Cravings	1	2	3	4	5
Energy	1	2	3	4	5
Mental Clarity	1	2	3	4	5
Stress	1	2	3	4	5
Sleep Quality	1	2	3	4	5

Fasting Stability Journal

Daily Tracking Day _____

Day: ____________________ Date: ____________________

5 Electrolytes / Fluids

Water ____________________

Sodium ____________________

Potassium ____________________

Magnesium ____________________

Caffeine ____________________

Exercise / Sweating ____________________

6 Notes / Observations

____

____

____

____

____

____

7 What Felt Stable?

____

____

____

____

8 What Felt Unstable?

____

____

____

____

____

Fasting Stability Journal

Daily Tracking Day ____

Day: ____________________ Date: ____________________

1 Fasting Window

Start: ______________ End: ______________ Total Hours: __________

2 Eating Window

Start: ____________________ End: ____________________

3 Morning Stats

Weight ____________________

Blood Glucose ____________________

Ketones ____________________

Blood Pressure ____________________

Resting Heart Rate ____________________

4 Daily Signals

Hunger	1	2	3	4	5
Cravings	1	2	3	4	5
Energy	1	2	3	4	5
Mental Clarity	1	2	3	4	5
Stress	1	2	3	4	5
Sleep Quality	1	2	3	4	5

Fasting Stability Journal

Daily Tracking Day _____

Day: ____________________ Date: ____________________

(5) Electrolytes / Fluids

Water ____________________

Sodium ____________________

Potassium ____________________

Magnesium ____________________

Caffeine ____________________

Exercise / Sweating ____________________

(6) Notes / Observations

____

____

____

____

____

____

(7) What Felt Stable?

____

____

____

____

(8) What Felt Unstable?

____

____

____

____

____

Fasting Stability Journal

Daily Tracking Day _____

Day: ______________________ Date: ______________________

1 Fasting Window

Start: ______________ End: ______________ Total Hours: __________

2 Eating Window

Start: ____________________ End: ________________

3 Morning Stats

Weight ____________________

Blood Glucose ________________

Ketones ____________________

Blood Pressure ________________

Resting Heart Rate ______________

4 Daily Signals

Hunger	1	2	3	4	5
Cravings	1	2	3	4	5
Energy	1	2	3	4	5
Mental Clarity	1	2	3	4	5
Stress	1	2	3	4	5
Sleep Quality	1	2	3	4	5

Fasting Stability Journal

Daily Tracking Day _____

Day: ____________________ Date: ____________________

(5) Electrolytes / Fluids

Water ____________________

Sodium ____________________

Potassium ____________________

Magnesium ____________________

Caffeine ____________________

Exercise / Sweating ____________________

(6) Notes / Observations

____

____

____

____

____

____

(7) What Felt Stable?

____

____

____

____

(8) What Felt Unstable?

____

____

____

____

____

Fasting Stability Journal

Daily Tracking Day _____

Day: ______________________ Date: ______________________

1 Fasting Window

Start: ______________ End: ______________ Total Hours: __________

2 Eating Window

Start: ______________________ End: ____________________

3 Morning Stats

Weight ______________________

Blood Glucose ________________

Ketones ______________________

Blood Pressure _______________

Resting Heart Rate ____________

4 Daily Signals

Hunger	1	2	3	4	5
Cravings	1	2	3	4	5
Energy	1	2	3	4	5
Mental Clarity	1	2	3	4	5
Stress	1	2	3	4	5
Sleep Quality	1	2	3	4	5

Fasting Stability Journal

Daily Tracking Day _____

Day: ____________________ Date: ____________________

(5) Electrolytes / Fluids

Water ____________________

Sodium ____________________

Potassium ____________________

Magnesium ____________________

Caffeine ____________________

Exercise / Sweating ____________________

(6) Notes / Observations

____

____

____

____

____

____

(7) What Felt Stable?

____

____

____

____

(8) What Felt Unstable?

____

____

____

____

____

Fasting Stability Journal

Weekly Review

1 Cycle Review

Cycle Start: ____________ Cycle End: ____________ Days Tracked: ________

2 Review Highlights

Most Stable Day: ____________________

Most Unstable Day: ____________________

Most Common Fasting Window: ____________________

Most Difficult Time of Day: ____________________

3 Signal Trends

Hunger	1	2	3	4	5
Cravings	1	2	3	4	5
Energy	1	2	3	4	5
Sleep	1	2	3	4	5
Stress	1	2	3	4	5

4 Main Patterns Noticed

____

____

____

____

5 What to Watch Next Cycle

____

____

____

____

____

Fasting Stability Journal

Daily Tracking Day ____

Day: ____________________ Date: ____________________

1 Fasting Window

Start: ______________ End: ______________ Total Hours: __________

2 Eating Window

Start: ____________________ End: ____________________

3 Morning Stats

Weight ____________________

Blood Glucose ________________

Ketones ____________________

Blood Pressure ________________

Resting Heart Rate ______________

4 Daily Signals

Hunger	1	2	3	4	5
Cravings	1	2	3	4	5
Energy	1	2	3	4	5
Mental Clarity	1	2	3	4	5
Stress	1	2	3	4	5
Sleep Quality	1	2	3	4	5

Fasting Stability Journal

Daily Tracking Day _____

Day: ____________________ Date: ____________________

(5) Electrolytes / Fluids

Water ______________________________

Sodium ______________________________

Potassium ______________________________

Magnesium ______________________________

Caffeine ______________________________

Exercise / Sweating ______________________________

(6) Notes / Observations

____

____

____

____

____

____

(7) What Felt Stable?

____

____

____

____

(8) What Felt Unstable?

____

____

____

____

____

Fasting Stability Journal

Daily Tracking Day _____

Day: ______________________ Date: ______________________

1 Fasting Window

Start: ______________ End: ______________ Total Hours: __________

2 Eating Window

Start: ______________________ End: ______________________

3 Morning Stats

Weight ______________________

Blood Glucose ______________________

Ketones ______________________

Blood Pressure ______________________

Resting Heart Rate ______________________

4 Daily Signals

Hunger	1	2	3	4	5
Cravings	1	2	3	4	5
Energy	1	2	3	4	5
Mental Clarity	1	2	3	4	5
Stress	1	2	3	4	5
Sleep Quality	1	2	3	4	5

Fasting Stability Journal

Daily Tracking Day _____

Day: ________________ Date: ________________

(5) Electrolytes / Fluids

Water ________________

Sodium ________________

Potassium ________________

Magnesium ________________

Caffeine ________________

Exercise / Sweating ________________

(6) Notes / Observations

____

____

____

____

____

____

(7) What Felt Stable?

____

____

____

____

(8) What Felt Unstable?

____

____

____

____

____

Fasting Stability Journal

Daily Tracking Day ____

Day: ______________ Date: ______________

1 Fasting Window

Start: ____________ End: ____________ Total Hours: ________

2 Eating Window

Start: ______________ End: ______________

3 Morning Stats

Weight ______________

Blood Glucose ______________

Ketones ______________

Blood Pressure ______________

Resting Heart Rate ______________

4 Daily Signals

Hunger	1	2	3	4	5
Cravings	1	2	3	4	5
Energy	1	2	3	4	5
Mental Clarity	1	2	3	4	5
Stress	1	2	3	4	5
Sleep Quality	1	2	3	4	5

Fasting Stability Journal

Daily Tracking Day _____

Day: ________________ Date: ________________

(5) Electrolytes / Fluids

Water ____________________

Sodium ____________________

Potassium ____________________

Magnesium ____________________

Caffeine ____________________

Exercise / Sweating ____________________

(6) Notes / Observations

(7) What Felt Stable?

(8) What Felt Unstable?

Fasting Stability Journal

Daily Tracking Day ____

Day: ______________________ **Date:** ______________________

① Fasting Window

Start: ______________ End: ______________ Total Hours: __________

② Eating Window

Start: ______________________ End: ______________________

③ Morning Stats

Weight ______________________

Blood Glucose ______________________

Ketones ______________________

Blood Pressure ______________________

Resting Heart Rate ______________________

④ Daily Signals

Hunger	1	2	3	4	5
Cravings	1	2	3	4	5
Energy	1	2	3	4	5
Mental Clarity	1	2	3	4	5
Stress	1	2	3	4	5
Sleep Quality	1	2	3	4	5

Fasting Stability Journal

Daily Tracking Day _____

Day: ____________________ Date: ____________________

5 Electrolytes / Fluids

Water ______________________________

Sodium ______________________________

Potassium ______________________________

Magnesium ______________________________

Caffeine ______________________________

Exercise / Sweating ______________________________

6 Notes / Observations

____

____

____

____

____

____

7 What Felt Stable?

____

____

____

____

8 What Felt Unstable?

____

____

____

____

____

Fasting Stability Journal

Daily Tracking Day ____

Day: ______________________ Date: ______________________

1 Fasting Window

Start: ______________ End: ______________ Total Hours: __________

2 Eating Window

Start: ______________________ End: ______________________

3 Morning Stats

Weight ______________________

Blood Glucose ______________________

Ketones ______________________

Blood Pressure ______________________

Resting Heart Rate ______________________

4 Daily Signals

Hunger	1	2	3	4	5
Cravings	1	2	3	4	5
Energy	1	2	3	4	5
Mental Clarity	1	2	3	4	5
Stress	1	2	3	4	5
Sleep Quality	1	2	3	4	5

Fasting Stability Journal

Daily Tracking Day _____

Day: ____________________ Date: ____________________

5 Electrolytes / Fluids

Water ____________________

Sodium ____________________

Potassium ____________________

Magnesium ____________________

Caffeine ____________________

Exercise / Sweating ____________________

6 Notes / Observations

7 What Felt Stable?

8 What Felt Unstable?

Fasting Stability Journal

Daily Tracking Day _____

Day: ______________________ Date: ______________________

1 Fasting Window

Start: ______________ End: ______________ Total Hours: __________

2 Eating Window

Start: ______________________ End: ______________________

3 Morning Stats

Weight ______________________

Blood Glucose ______________________

Ketones ______________________

Blood Pressure ______________________

Resting Heart Rate ______________________

4 Daily Signals

Hunger	1	2	3	4	5
Cravings	1	2	3	4	5
Energy	1	2	3	4	5
Mental Clarity	1	2	3	4	5
Stress	1	2	3	4	5
Sleep Quality	1	2	3	4	5

Fasting Stability Journal

Daily Tracking Day _____

Day: ____________________ Date: ____________________

5 Electrolytes / Fluids

Water ____________________

Sodium ____________________

Potassium ____________________

Magnesium ____________________

Caffeine ____________________

Exercise / Sweating ____________________

6 Notes / Observations

7 What Felt Stable?

8 What Felt Unstable?

Fasting Stability Journal

Daily Tracking Day ____

Day: ______________________ **Date:** ______________________

① Fasting Window

Start: ______________ End: ______________ Total Hours: __________

② Eating Window

Start: ______________________ End: ______________________

③ Morning Stats

Weight ______________________

Blood Glucose ______________________

Ketones ______________________

Blood Pressure ______________________

Resting Heart Rate ______________________

④ Daily Signals

Hunger	1	2	3	4	5
Cravings	1	2	3	4	5
Energy	1	2	3	4	5
Mental Clarity	1	2	3	4	5
Stress	1	2	3	4	5
Sleep Quality	1	2	3	4	5

Fasting Stability Journal

Daily Tracking Day _____

Day: ________________ Date: ________________

⑤ Electrolytes / Fluids

Water ____________________

Sodium ____________________

Potassium ____________________

Magnesium ____________________

Caffeine ____________________

Exercise / Sweating ____________________

⑥ Notes / Observations

⑦ What Felt Stable?

⑧ What Felt Unstable?

Fasting Stability Journal

Weekly Review

1 Cycle Review

Cycle Start: ____________ Cycle End: ____________ Days Tracked: ________

2 Review Highlights

Most Stable Day: ____________________

Most Unstable Day: ____________________

Most Common Fasting Window: ____________________

Most Difficult Time of Day: ____________________

3 Signal Trends

Hunger	1	2	3	4	5
Cravings	1	2	3	4	5
Energy	1	2	3	4	5
Sleep	1	2	3	4	5
Stress	1	2	3	4	5

4 Main Patterns Noticed

____

____

____

____

5 What to Watch Next Cycle

____

____

____

____

____

Fasting Stability Journal

Daily Tracking Day _____

Day: ____________________ Date: ____________________

1 Fasting Window

Start: ______________ End: ____________ Total Hours: ________

2 Eating Window

Start: ____________________ End: ________________

3 Morning Stats

Weight ________________

Blood Glucose ______________

Ketones ________________

Blood Pressure ______________

Resting Heart Rate ____________

4 Daily Signals

Hunger	1	2	3	4	5
Cravings	1	2	3	4	5
Energy	1	2	3	4	5
Mental Clarity	1	2	3	4	5
Stress	1	2	3	4	5
Sleep Quality	1	2	3	4	5

Fasting Stability Journal

Daily Tracking Day _____

Day: ____________________ Date: ____________________

(5) Electrolytes / Fluids

Water ____________________

Sodium ____________________

Potassium ____________________

Magnesium ____________________

Caffeine ____________________

Exercise / Sweating ____________________

(6) Notes / Observations

____

____

____

____

____

____

(7) What Felt Stable?

____

____

____

____

(8) What Felt Unstable?

____

____

____

____

____

Fasting Stability Journal

Daily Tracking Day ____

Day: ______________________ Date: ______________________

1 Fasting Window

Start: ______________ End: ____________ Total Hours: ________

2 Eating Window

Start: ____________________ End: ________________

3 Morning Stats

Weight ____________________

Blood Glucose ________________

Ketones ____________________

Blood Pressure ________________

Resting Heart Rate ______________

4 Daily Signals

Hunger	1	2	3	4	5
Cravings	1	2	3	4	5
Energy	1	2	3	4	5
Mental Clarity	1	2	3	4	5
Stress	1	2	3	4	5
Sleep Quality	1	2	3	4	5

Fasting Stability Journal

Daily Tracking Day _____

Day: ____________________ Date: ____________________

⑤ Electrolytes / Fluids

Water ____________________

Sodium ____________________

Potassium ____________________

Magnesium ____________________

Caffeine ____________________

Exercise / Sweating ____________________

⑥ Notes / Observations

⑦ What Felt Stable?

⑧ What Felt Unstable?

Fasting Stability Journal

Daily Tracking Day ____

Day: ______________ Date: ______________

1 Fasting Window

Start: __________ End: __________ Total Hours: __________

2 Eating Window

Start: __________ End: __________

3 Morning Stats

Weight __________

Blood Glucose __________

Ketones __________

Blood Pressure __________

Resting Heart Rate __________

4 Daily Signals

Hunger	1	2	3	4	5
Cravings	1	2	3	4	5
Energy	1	2	3	4	5
Mental Clarity	1	2	3	4	5
Stress	1	2	3	4	5
Sleep Quality	1	2	3	4	5

Fasting Stability Journal

Daily Tracking Day _____

Day: ____________________ Date: ____________________

(5) Electrolytes / Fluids

Water ____________________

Sodium ____________________

Potassium ____________________

Magnesium ____________________

Caffeine ____________________

Exercise / Sweating ____________________

(6) Notes / Observations

____

____

____

____

____

____

(7) What Felt Stable?

____

____

____

____

(8) What Felt Unstable?

____

____

____

____

____

Fasting Stability Journal

Daily Tracking Day ____

Day: ______________________ **Date:** ______________________

1 Fasting Window

Start: ________________ End: ______________ Total Hours: __________

2 Eating Window

Start: ______________________ End: ________________

3 Morning Stats

Weight ______________________

Blood Glucose ________________

Ketones ______________________

Blood Pressure ________________

Resting Heart Rate ______________

4 Daily Signals

Hunger	1	2	3	4	5
Cravings	1	2	3	4	5
Energy	1	2	3	4	5
Mental Clarity	1	2	3	4	5
Stress	1	2	3	4	5
Sleep Quality	1	2	3	4	5

Fasting Stability Journal

Daily Tracking Day _____

Day: ____________________ Date: ____________________

5 Electrolytes / Fluids

Water ____________________

Sodium ____________________

Potassium ____________________

Magnesium ____________________

Caffeine ____________________

Exercise / Sweating ____________________

6 Notes / Observations

____

____

____

____

____

____

7 What Felt Stable?

____

____

____

____

8 What Felt Unstable?

____

____

____

____

____

Fasting Stability Journal

Daily Tracking Day ____

Day: ____________________ Date: ____________________

① Fasting Window

Start: ______________ End: ______________ Total Hours: ________

② Eating Window

Start: ____________________ End: ________________

③ Morning Stats

Weight ____________________

Blood Glucose ________________

Ketones ____________________

Blood Pressure ________________

Resting Heart Rate ______________

④ Daily Signals

Hunger	1	2	3	4	5
Cravings	1	2	3	4	5
Energy	1	2	3	4	5
Mental Clarity	1	2	3	4	5
Stress	1	2	3	4	5
Sleep Quality	1	2	3	4	5

Fasting Stability Journal

Daily Tracking Day _____

Day: ____________________ Date: ____________________

⑤ Electrolytes / Fluids

Water ____________________

Sodium ____________________

Potassium ____________________

Magnesium ____________________

Caffeine ____________________

Exercise / Sweating ____________________

⑥ Notes / Observations

____

____

____

____

____

____

⑦ What Felt Stable?

____

____

____

____

⑧ What Felt Unstable?

____

____

____

____

____

Fasting Stability Journal

Daily Tracking Day _____

Day: ______________________ Date: ______________________

1 Fasting Window

Start: ______________ End: ______________ Total Hours: __________

2 Eating Window

Start: ______________________ End: ______________________

3 Morning Stats

Weight ______________________

Blood Glucose ______________________

Ketones ______________________

Blood Pressure ______________________

Resting Heart Rate ______________________

4 Daily Signals

Hunger	1	2	3	4	5
Cravings	1	2	3	4	5
Energy	1	2	3	4	5
Mental Clarity	1	2	3	4	5
Stress	1	2	3	4	5
Sleep Quality	1	2	3	4	5

Fasting Stability Journal

Daily Tracking Day _____

Day: ____________________ Date: ____________________

(5) Electrolytes / Fluids

Water ____________________

Sodium ____________________

Potassium ____________________

Magnesium ____________________

Caffeine ____________________

Exercise / Sweating ____________________

(6) Notes / Observations

____

____

____

____

____

____

(7) What Felt Stable?

____

____

____

____

(8) What Felt Unstable?

____

____

____

____

____

Fasting Stability Journal

Daily Tracking Day _____

Day: ____________________ Date: ____________________

1 Fasting Window

Start: ______________ End: ______________ Total Hours: __________

2 Eating Window

Start: ____________________ End: ______________

3 Morning Stats

Weight ____________________

Blood Glucose ______________

Ketones ____________________

Blood Pressure ______________

Resting Heart Rate ______________

4 Daily Signals

Hunger	1	2	3	4	5
Cravings	1	2	3	4	5
Energy	1	2	3	4	5
Mental Clarity	1	2	3	4	5
Stress	1	2	3	4	5
Sleep Quality	1	2	3	4	5

Fasting Stability Journal

Daily Tracking Day _____

Day: ____________________ Date: ____________________

5 Electrolytes / Fluids

Water ____________________

Sodium ____________________

Potassium ____________________

Magnesium ____________________

Caffeine ____________________

Exercise / Sweating ____________________

6 Notes / Observations

7 What Felt Stable?

8 What Felt Unstable?

Fasting Stability Journal

Weekly Review

1 Cycle Review

Cycle Start: ____________ Cycle End: ____________ Days Tracked: ________

2 Review Highlights

Most Stable Day: ____________

Most Unstable Day: ____________

Most Common Fasting Window: ____________

Most Difficult Time of Day: ____________

3 Signal Trends

Hunger	1	2	3	4	5
Cravings	1	2	3	4	5
Energy	1	2	3	4	5
Sleep	1	2	3	4	5
Stress	1	2	3	4	5

4 Main Patterns Noticed

____

____

____

____

5 What to Watch Next Cycle

____

____

____

____

____

Fasting Stability Journal

Daily Tracking Day _____

Day: ______________________ **Date:** ______________________

(1) Fasting Window

Start: ______________ End: ______________ Total Hours: __________

(2) Eating Window

Start: ______________________ End: ______________________

(3) Morning Stats

Weight ______________________

Blood Glucose ______________________

Ketones ______________________

Blood Pressure ______________________

Resting Heart Rate ______________________

(4) Daily Signals

Hunger	1	2	3	4	5
Cravings	1	2	3	4	5
Energy	1	2	3	4	5
Mental Clarity	1	2	3	4	5
Stress	1	2	3	4	5
Sleep Quality	1	2	3	4	5

Fasting Stability Journal

Daily Tracking Day _____

Day: ____________________ Date: ____________________

5 Electrolytes / Fluids

Water ____________________

Sodium ____________________

Potassium ____________________

Magnesium ____________________

Caffeine ____________________

Exercise / Sweating ____________________

6 Notes / Observations

7 What Felt Stable?

8 What Felt Unstable?

Fasting Stability Journal

Daily Tracking Day _____

Day: ______________________ Date: ______________________

1 Fasting Window

Start: ______________ End: ______________ Total Hours: __________

2 Eating Window

Start: ______________________ End: ______________________

3 Morning Stats

Weight ______________________

Blood Glucose ______________________

Ketones ______________________

Blood Pressure ______________________

Resting Heart Rate ______________________

4 Daily Signals

Hunger	1	2	3	4	5
Cravings	1	2	3	4	5
Energy	1	2	3	4	5
Mental Clarity	1	2	3	4	5
Stress	1	2	3	4	5
Sleep Quality	1	2	3	4	5

Fasting Stability Journal

Daily Tracking Day _____

Day: ____________________ Date: ____________________

5 Electrolytes / Fluids

Water ____________________

Sodium ____________________

Potassium ____________________

Magnesium ____________________

Caffeine ____________________

Exercise / Sweating ____________________

6 Notes / Observations

____

____

____

____

____

____

7 What Felt Stable?

____

____

____

____

8 What Felt Unstable?

____

____

____

____

____

Fasting Stability Journal

Daily Tracking Day ____

Day: ____________________ Date: ____________________

1 Fasting Window

Start: ______________ End: ____________ Total Hours: ________

2 Eating Window

Start: ____________________ End: ________________

3 Morning Stats

Weight ________________

Blood Glucose ______________

Ketones ________________

Blood Pressure ______________

Resting Heart Rate ____________

4 Daily Signals

Hunger	1	2	3	4	5
Cravings	1	2	3	4	5
Energy	1	2	3	4	5
Mental Clarity	1	2	3	4	5
Stress	1	2	3	4	5
Sleep Quality	1	2	3	4	5

Fasting Stability Journal

Daily Tracking Day _____

Day: ____________________ Date: ____________________

(5) Electrolytes / Fluids

Water ____________________

Sodium ____________________

Potassium ____________________

Magnesium ____________________

Caffeine ____________________

Exercise / Sweating ____________________

(6) Notes / Observations

____

____

____

____

____

____

(7) What Felt Stable?

____

____

____

____

(8) What Felt Unstable?

____

____

____

____

____

Fasting Stability Journal

Daily Tracking Day _____

Day: ____________________ Date: ____________________

1 Fasting Window

Start: ______________ End: ____________ Total Hours: ________

2 Eating Window

Start: ____________________ End: ________________

3 Morning Stats

Weight ____________________

Blood Glucose ________________

Ketones ____________________

Blood Pressure ________________

Resting Heart Rate ______________

4 Daily Signals

Hunger	1	2	3	4	5
Cravings	1	2	3	4	5
Energy	1	2	3	4	5
Mental Clarity	1	2	3	4	5
Stress	1	2	3	4	5
Sleep Quality	1	2	3	4	5

Fasting Stability Journal

Daily Tracking Day _____

Day: ____________________ Date: ____________________

5 Electrolytes / Fluids

Water ____________________

Sodium ____________________

Potassium ____________________

Magnesium ____________________

Caffeine ____________________

Exercise / Sweating ____________________

6 Notes / Observations

7 What Felt Stable?

8 What Felt Unstable?

Fasting Stability Journal

Daily Tracking Day _____

Day: ____________________ Date: ____________________

① Fasting Window

Start: ______________ End: ______________ Total Hours: __________

② Eating Window

Start: ____________________ End: ______________

③ Morning Stats

Weight ____________________

Blood Glucose ______________

Ketones ____________________

Blood Pressure ______________

Resting Heart Rate ______________

④ Daily Signals

Hunger	1	2	3	4	5
Cravings	1	2	3	4	5
Energy	1	2	3	4	5
Mental Clarity	1	2	3	4	5
Stress	1	2	3	4	5
Sleep Quality	1	2	3	4	5

Fasting Stability Journal

Daily Tracking Day _____

Day: ________________ Date: ________________

⑤ Electrolytes / Fluids

Water ______________________________

Sodium ______________________________

Potassium ______________________________

Magnesium ______________________________

Caffeine ______________________________

Exercise / Sweating ______________________________

⑥ Notes / Observations

____

____

____

____

____

____

⑦ What Felt Stable?

____

____

____

____

⑧ What Felt Unstable?

____

____

____

____

____

Fasting Stability Journal

Daily Tracking Day ____

Day: ______________________ Date: ______________________

1 Fasting Window

Start: ______________ End: ______________ Total Hours: ________

2 Eating Window

Start: ____________________ End: ________________

3 Morning Stats

Weight ____________________

Blood Glucose ________________

Ketones ____________________

Blood Pressure ________________

Resting Heart Rate ______________

4 Daily Signals

Hunger	1	2	3	4	5
Cravings	1	2	3	4	5
Energy	1	2	3	4	5
Mental Clarity	1	2	3	4	5
Stress	1	2	3	4	5
Sleep Quality	1	2	3	4	5

Fasting Stability Journal

Daily Tracking Day _____

Day: ____________________ Date: ____________________

(5) Electrolytes / Fluids

Water ____________________

Sodium ____________________

Potassium ____________________

Magnesium ____________________

Caffeine ____________________

Exercise / Sweating ____________________

(6) Notes / Observations

____

____

____

____

____

____

(7) What Felt Stable?

____

____

____

____

(8) What Felt Unstable?

____

____

____

____

____

Fasting Stability Journal

Daily Tracking Day _____

Day: ____________________ Date: ____________________

1 Fasting Window

Start: ______________ End: ______________ Total Hours: __________

2 Eating Window

Start: ____________________ End: ________________

3 Morning Stats

Weight ____________________

Blood Glucose ________________

Ketones ____________________

Blood Pressure ________________

Resting Heart Rate ______________

4 Daily Signals

Hunger	1	2	3	4	5
Cravings	1	2	3	4	5
Energy	1	2	3	4	5
Mental Clarity	1	2	3	4	5
Stress	1	2	3	4	5
Sleep Quality	1	2	3	4	5

Fasting Stability Journal

Daily Tracking Day _____

Day: ____________________ Date: ____________________

(5) Electrolytes / Fluids

Water ____________________

Sodium ____________________

Potassium ____________________

Magnesium ____________________

Caffeine ____________________

Exercise / Sweating ____________________

(6) Notes / Observations

____

____

____

____

____

____

(7) What Felt Stable?

____

____

____

____

(8) What Felt Unstable?

____

____

____

____

____

Fasting Stability Journal

Weekly Review

1 Cycle Review

Cycle Start: ____________ Cycle End: ____________ Days Tracked: ________

2 Review Highlights

Most Stable Day: ____________________

Most Unstable Day: ____________________

Most Common Fasting Window: ____________________

Most Difficult Time of Day: ____________________

3 Signal Trends

Hunger	1	2	3	4	5
Cravings	1	2	3	4	5
Energy	1	2	3	4	5
Sleep	1	2	3	4	5
Stress	1	2	3	4	5

4 Main Patterns Noticed

____

____

____

____

5 What to Watch Next Cycle

____

____

____

____

____

Fasting Stability Journal

Daily Tracking Day ____

Day: ____________________ Date: ____________________

1 Fasting Window

Start: ______________ End: ____________ Total Hours: ________

2 Eating Window

Start: ____________________ End: ________________

3 Morning Stats

Weight ____________________

Blood Glucose ______________

Ketones ____________________

Blood Pressure ______________

Resting Heart Rate ____________

4 Daily Signals

Hunger	1	2	3	4	5
Cravings	1	2	3	4	5
Energy	1	2	3	4	5
Mental Clarity	1	2	3	4	5
Stress	1	2	3	4	5
Sleep Quality	1	2	3	4	5

Fasting Stability Journal

Daily Tracking Day _____

Day: ____________________ Date: ____________________

(5) Electrolytes / Fluids

Water ____________________

Sodium ____________________

Potassium ____________________

Magnesium ____________________

Caffeine ____________________

Exercise / Sweating ____________________

(6) Notes / Observations

____

____

____

____

____

____

(7) What Felt Stable?

____

____

____

____

(8) What Felt Unstable?

____

____

____

____

____

Fasting Stability Journal

Daily Tracking Day _____

Day: ____________________ Date: ____________________

1 Fasting Window

Start: ____________ End: ____________ Total Hours: ________

2 Eating Window

Start: ____________________ End: ____________________

3 Morning Stats

Weight ____________________

Blood Glucose ____________________

Ketones ____________________

Blood Pressure ____________________

Resting Heart Rate ____________________

4 Daily Signals

Hunger	1	2	3	4	5
Cravings	1	2	3	4	5
Energy	1	2	3	4	5
Mental Clarity	1	2	3	4	5
Stress	1	2	3	4	5
Sleep Quality	1	2	3	4	5

Fasting Stability Journal

Daily Tracking Day _____

Day: ____________________ Date: ____________________

5 Electrolytes / Fluids

Water ____________________

Sodium ____________________

Potassium ____________________

Magnesium ____________________

Caffeine ____________________

Exercise / Sweating ____________________

6 Notes / Observations

7 What Felt Stable?

8 What Felt Unstable?

Fasting Stability Journal

Daily Tracking Day _____

Day: ____________________ Date: ____________________

1 Fasting Window

Start: ______________ End: ______________ Total Hours: __________

2 Eating Window

Start: ____________________ End: ________________

3 Morning Stats

Weight ____________________

Blood Glucose ________________

Ketones ____________________

Blood Pressure ________________

Resting Heart Rate ______________

4 Daily Signals

Hunger	1	2	3	4	5
Cravings	1	2	3	4	5
Energy	1	2	3	4	5
Mental Clarity	1	2	3	4	5
Stress	1	2	3	4	5
Sleep Quality	1	2	3	4	5

Fasting Stability Journal

Daily Tracking Day _____

Day: ____________________ Date: ____________________

⑤ Electrolytes / Fluids

Water ____________________

Sodium ____________________

Potassium ____________________

Magnesium ____________________

Caffeine ____________________

Exercise / Sweating ____________________

⑥ Notes / Observations

⑦ What Felt Stable?

⑧ What Felt Unstable?

Fasting Stability Journal

Daily Tracking Day ____

Day: ______________________ Date: ______________________

1 Fasting Window

Start: ______________ End: ______________ Total Hours: __________

2 Eating Window

Start: ______________________ End: ________________

3 Morning Stats

Weight ______________________

Blood Glucose ________________

Ketones ______________________

Blood Pressure ________________

Resting Heart Rate ______________

4 Daily Signals

Hunger	1	2	3	4	5
Cravings	1	2	3	4	5
Energy	1	2	3	4	5
Mental Clarity	1	2	3	4	5
Stress	1	2	3	4	5
Sleep Quality	1	2	3	4	5

Fasting Stability Journal

Daily Tracking Day _____

Day: ____________________ Date: ____________________

(5) Electrolytes / Fluids

Water ____________________

Sodium ____________________

Potassium ____________________

Magnesium ____________________

Caffeine ____________________

Exercise / Sweating ____________________

(6) Notes / Observations

(7) What Felt Stable?

(8) What Felt Unstable?

Fasting Stability Journal

Daily Tracking Day _____

Day: ______________________ Date: ______________________

① Fasting Window

Start: ______________ End: ______________ Total Hours: __________

② Eating Window

Start: ______________________ End: ______________________

③ Morning Stats

Weight ______________________

Blood Glucose ______________________

Ketones ______________________

Blood Pressure ______________________

Resting Heart Rate ______________________

④ Daily Signals

Hunger	1	2	3	4	5
Cravings	1	2	3	4	5
Energy	1	2	3	4	5
Mental Clarity	1	2	3	4	5
Stress	1	2	3	4	5
Sleep Quality	1	2	3	4	5

Fasting Stability Journal

Daily Tracking Day _____

Day: ____________________ Date: ____________________

5 Electrolytes / Fluids

Water ____________________

Sodium ____________________

Potassium ____________________

Magnesium ____________________

Caffeine ____________________

Exercise / Sweating ____________________

6 Notes / Observations

7 What Felt Stable?

8 What Felt Unstable?

Fasting Stability Journal

Daily Tracking Day ____

Day: ______________________ Date: ______________________

1 Fasting Window

Start: ________________ End: ______________ Total Hours: __________

2 Eating Window

Start: ______________________ End: __________________

3 Morning Stats

Weight ____________________

Blood Glucose ________________

Ketones ____________________

Blood Pressure ________________

Resting Heart Rate ______________

4 Daily Signals

Hunger	1	2	3	4	5
Cravings	1	2	3	4	5
Energy	1	2	3	4	5
Mental Clarity	1	2	3	4	5
Stress	1	2	3	4	5
Sleep Quality	1	2	3	4	5

Fasting Stability Journal

Daily Tracking Day _____

Day: ____________ Date: ____________

(5) Electrolytes / Fluids

Water ____________

Sodium ____________

Potassium ____________

Magnesium ____________

Caffeine ____________

Exercise / Sweating ____________

(6) Notes / Observations

(7) What Felt Stable?

(8) What Felt Unstable?

Fasting Stability Journal

Daily Tracking Day ____

Day: ____________________ **Date:** ____________________

① Fasting Window

Start: ______________ End: ______________ Total Hours: ________

② Eating Window

Start: ____________________ End: ______________

③ Morning Stats

Weight ____________________

Blood Glucose ______________

Ketones ____________________

Blood Pressure ______________

Resting Heart Rate ____________

④ Daily Signals

Hunger	1	2	3	4	5
Cravings	1	2	3	4	5
Energy	1	2	3	4	5
Mental Clarity	1	2	3	4	5
Stress	1	2	3	4	5
Sleep Quality	1	2	3	4	5

Fasting Stability Journal

Daily Tracking Day _____

Day: ____________________ Date: ____________________

5 Electrolytes / Fluids

Water ____________________

Sodium ____________________

Potassium ____________________

Magnesium ____________________

Caffeine ____________________

Exercise / Sweating ____________________

6 Notes / Observations

7 What Felt Stable?

8 What Felt Unstable?

After the Fast

12-WEEK REVIEW

Weeks ________ to ________ Date ____________

1. OVERALL PROGRESS

How would I describe my progress over this 12-week period?

2. BIGGEST WINS	2. BIGGEST CHALLENGES
What are my top 3 wins?	What were my biggest challenges?
1. ____________	1. ____________
2. ____________	2. ____________
3. ____________	3. ____________

3. WHAT I'VE LEARNED

Key lessons from this 12-week period.

4. NEXT 12 WEEKS FOCUS

What I will focus on next.

Fasting Stability Journal

Hunger / Craving Pattern Notes

1 Hunger Timing

When hunger appeared most often: ______________________________

When hunger felt most intense: ______________________________

When hunger felt least intense: ______________________________

2 Craving Pattern

When cravings appeared most often: ______________________________

What cravings were linked to: ______________________________

Did intensity rise, fall, or repeat: ______________________________

3 Trigger Context

- ☐ Timing
- ☐ Stress
- ☐ Fatigue
- ☐ Habit
- ☐ Environment
- ☐ Poor Sleep
- ☐ Social Cues
- ☐ Other: ______________________

4 What Reduced Amplification?

____

____

____

____

5 Additional Notes

____

____

____

____

Fasting Stability Journal

Energy / Recovery Pattern Notes

1 Energy Pattern

When energy felt most stable: ____________________

When energy dipped or crashed: ____________________

Most common energy pattern noticed: ____________________

2 Recovery Pattern

How sleep affected the fast: ____________________

How activity or training affected recovery: ____________________

How work or stress affected recovery: ____________________

3 Influences to Watch

- ☐ Sleep
- ☐ Stress
- ☐ Training
- ☐ Workload
- ☐ Travel
- ☐ Fasting Duration
- ☐ Electrolytes / Fluids
- ☐ Other: ____________________

4 What Helped Recovery?

____

____

____

____

5 Additional Notes

____

____

____

____

____

Fasting Stability Journal

Electrolyte / Fluid Notes

1 Hydration Pattern

What hydration felt like: ______________________________

When fluids felt most needed: ______________________________

Most common hydration pattern noticed: ______________________________

2 Electrolyte Pattern

What electrolyte support was used: ______________________________

When electrolytes felt most needed: ______________________________

Most common electrolyte pattern noticed: ______________________________

3 Signals Noticed

- [ ] Headache
- [ ] Lightheadedness
- [ ] Fatigue
- [ ] Thirst
- [ ] Cramps
- [ ] Brain Fog
- [ ] Weakness
- [ ] Other: ______________

4 What Seemed to Help?

____

____

____

____

5 Additional Notes

____

____

____

____

Fasting Stability Journal

Sleep / Stress Notes

1 Sleep Pattern

When sleep felt most supportive: ____________________

When sleep felt least supportive: ____________________

Most common sleep pattern noticed: ____________________

2 Stress Pattern

When stress felt highest: ____________________

When stress seemed to affect the fast most: ____________________

Most common stress pattern noticed: ____________________

3 Influences to Watch

- ☐ Workload
- ☐ Travel
- ☐ Poor Routine
- ☐ Training
- ☐ Poor Recovery
- ☐ Social Load
- ☐ Mental Load
- ☐ Other: ____________________

4 What Increased Stability?

____

____

____

____

5 Additional Notes

____

____

____

____

____

Fasting Stability Journal

What Remained Stable?

1 Stable Signals

- [ ] Hunger
- [ ] Cravings
- [ ] Energy
- [ ] Sleep
- [ ] Stress
- [ ] Focus
- [ ] Mood
- [ ] Hydration
- [ ] Electrolytes
- [ ] Recovery

2 Stable Patterns

3 Stable Routines

4 What Supported Stability?

5 Additional Notes

Fasting Stability Journal

What Changed?

1 Changed Signals

- [ ] Hunger
- [ ] Cravings
- [ ] Energy
- [ ] Sleep
- [ ] Stress
- [ ] Focus
- [ ] Mood
- [ ] Hydration
- [ ] Electrolytes
- [ ] Recovery

2 Changed Patterns

3 Changed Routines

4 What Seemed to Shift Most?

5 Additional Notes

Fasting Stability Journal

Next Fasting Cycle Plan

1 Next Cycle Details

Planned Start Date: ____________________

Planned Duration: ____________________

Main Focus: ____________________

2 What to Repeat

3 What to Watch More Closely

4 What to Avoid Forcing

5 Questions for the Next Cycle

Fasting Stability Journal

Notes

1. General Notes

2. Observations

3. Questions

4. Additional Notes

Fasting Journal Series

The Fasting Stability Journal line is designed for different tracking cycles.

Some readers may want a short fasting record for a single week. Others may want a longer journal for a month, a full season, or a complete 90-day cycle. Each journal uses the same basic tracking system so fasting windows, eating windows, hunger, cravings, energy, electrolytes, fluids, sleep, stress, and recovery can be recorded consistently over time.

Available and planned journals include:

7-Day Fasting Journal

A short guided tracker for a single fasting cycle, reset, or observation week.

14-Day Fasting Journal

A two-week tracker for readers who want a slightly longer fasting record without committing to a full month.

30-Day Fasting Journal

A practical monthly journal for tracking fasting patterns, appetite signals, energy, sleep, electrolytes, and recovery across a longer cycle.

12-Week Fasting Journal

A full-season tracking journal designed for readers who want to observe patterns over several weeks.

90-Day Fasting Journal

A quarterly fasting journal for longer observation cycles and repeat use throughout the year.

The Fasting Journal Guide

A companion guide explaining how to use the journals, read fasting signals, review patterns, and keep tracking observational rather than rigid.

These journals are not fasting protocols, diet plans, or medical programs. They are guided tracking tools for recording patterns, reviewing signals, and understanding how fasting feels across different contexts.

More from Nathan Reed

Nathan Reed's books explain fasting, metabolism, appetite, energy, glucose, insulin, recovery, and long-term metabolic function through a systems-based lens.

For readers who want more context behind the patterns tracked in this journal, related titles include:

Fasting Fundamentals

A clear introduction to fasting, fasting windows, hunger, energy, electrolytes, and recovery.

Intermittent Fasting

A focused guide to daily fasting windows, feeding patterns, appetite rhythm, and metabolic response.

Prolonged Fasting

A deeper look at longer fasting windows, adaptation, electrolytes, recovery, and system strain.

Electrolytes

A focused guide to sodium, potassium, magnesium, hydration, fasting, exercise, and recovery.

Metabolic Stability

A systems guide to blood sugar, fasting, and long-term metabolic health.

Energy Stability

A guide to fuel, fatigue, recovery, and daily function.

Blood Sugar Stability

A guide to glucose fluctuations, insulin signals, and metabolic regulation.

Bulk and Institutional Orders

For bulk or institutional orders, contact Perennial Publishing at: orders@perennialpublishing.org

This journal may be useful for wellness groups, fasting education programs, coaching environments, workplace wellness initiatives, clinics, health educators, and structured self-tracking groups that want a simple fasting observation tool.

This journal is not a medical protocol, diet plan, or treatment guide. It is designed as a personal tracking and reflection tool.

Made in the USA
Monee, IL
04 November 2026

67382289R00125